Published by Herbivore Books.

www.bonzaiaphrodite.com
www.herbivoreclothing.com

Printed in the United States of America.

ISBN 978-0-9801440-3-1

Cover and illustrations by Leslie R. Magee

First edition 2011
Second edition 2013
Third edition 2014

For all my many mothers, here and gone:
Heidi, Shira, Barbara, and Lisa.

A huge and heartfelt thank you to

Matthew Ruscigno, MPH, RD, for lending your expertise in all things nutrition-related. This book wouldn't have been complete without your invaluable input . . . and your professional blessing. Thank you!

And very special thanks to some amazing women – Linda, Kim, Monika, Krysta, Leigh, Steph, Michelle, Angela, Katie, Lenn, and too many more to name. Thank you for your precious, priceless wisdom.

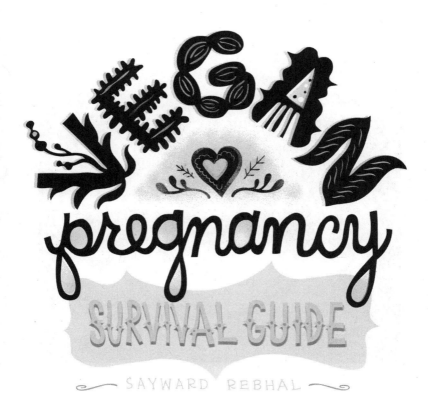

VEGAN pregnancy SURVIVAL GUIDE

SAYWARD REBHAL

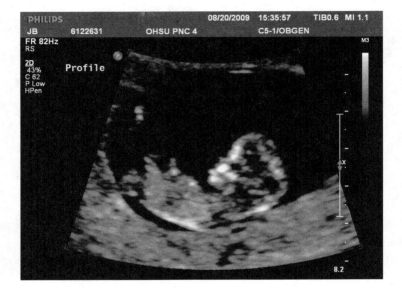

Table of Contents

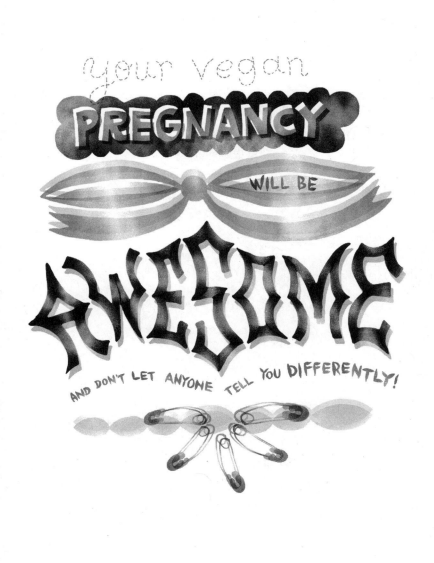

your vegan
PREGNANCY
WILL BE
AWESOME
AND DON'T LET ANYONE TELL YOU DIFFERENTLY!

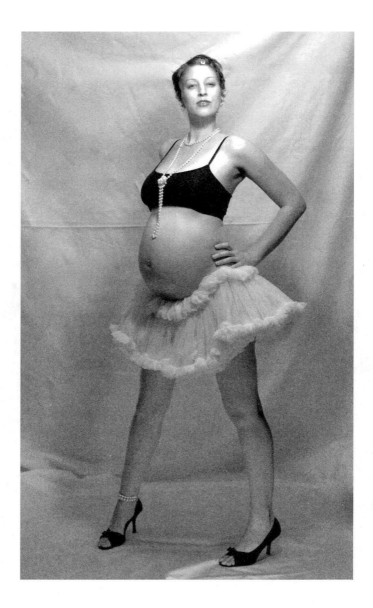

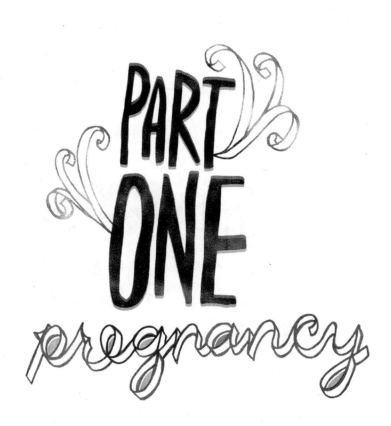

PART
ONE
pregnancy

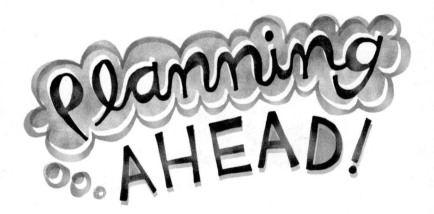

Congratulations! You're about to embark on a truly amazing journey, and I'm just tickled that I get to be here to help you along. If this is your first pregnancy: welcome to the wildest ride you've known. If this is your first *vegan* pregnancy, well then hey there mama! I'm so happy to see you here.

☞ My Promise #1 - Things can get pretty complicated.

☞ My Promise #2 - It's gonna be _so_ _much_ _fun!_

But it can also be pretty daunting. And crazy-making…and overwhelming. One of the best ways to maximize the fun and to minimize the madness, is to always stay a step ahead. The advice in this chapter is aimed at helping you to do just that. It's best to begin it before you're pregnant, but if that's not an option (Yay! Congrats!) just start as soon as you're able. That's ASAP. The quicker you get this stuff taken care of, the smoother this wild ride will be. Buckle up.

Quit Smoking; Cut Down On Caffeine; Nix Toxic Foods
All your conventional pregnancy books will cover these important points, so I'll spare you the lecture and keep it brief.

1) Yes, please quit smoking - <u>all the way!</u> I was a smoker for 12+ years and I quit a year and a half before getting pregnant. It was the hardest thing I've ever done. It took me an entire year to completely disentangle myself from cigarettes. *But,* now that I'm on the other side I can assure you that it's worth the work. Every second of soul-sucking suckiness was worth the freedom I get to feel now. It was *definitely* worth my peace of mind during pregnancy. But enough of that. You don't need me to tell you what you already know. Just get on it!

2) And now for some good news: caffeine is not, actually, The Devil. It certainly ain't health food, but in true moderation it can have an appropriate place in pregnancy. I personally quit caffeine completely when I got pregnant. Cold Tofurkey. It caused a 3-day-long headache and then that was the end of that. But, if you just can't imagine going without, try to cut back to one dose a day.[1][2] Savor your morning ritual and make that single serving really, *really* good.

3) Food matters. Consider that this is something you're doing at least three times a day, every single day. It has to have an impact! Your good health is in your control; you have all the power. How cool is that? We'll get into the nitty gritty of nutrition in the next chapter, but suffice it to say: cut the sugar and sugary drinks, cut the booze and processed foods, and cut the artificial *everythings* (sweeteners, colorings, flavors).

Start Your Prenatal Vitamins
Many women wait until they're already cooking their bun, but the truth is that you need those extra nutrients before you

even conceive.[3][4][5] You want to begin the baby building with all your stores at max capacity. Luckily there's plenty of vegan options out there, like Rainbow Light's Prenatal One™, which is food-based and widely available in many mainstream drugstores. I like to use the prenatal from Deva, an all-vegan company. Garden of Life Vitamin Code has claimed to be vegan, but is not.[6][7]

Find A Veg-Friendly Prenatal Care Provider

Doctors are not dieticians, and unfortunately many of them have antiquated ideas about nutrition. The same is true of midwives. You'd think that the crunchier folk would be more open-minded, but alas when it comes to food, the hippies are often just as traditional. One of the women I interviewed had a naturopathic midwife give her a heartburn aid made from pig's stomach. In her own words, "Ew."

So shop around, and make sure you find someone who supports a vegan lifestyle. They don't have to be an herbivore too, but they do have to be familiar with the basics of plant-based nutrition. Most importantly, make sure that they respect your decision to remain vegan. Pregnancy may put you into various vulnerable positions. You need to partner with somebody who you can trust, *not* somebody who would push red meat if your iron levels dipped. Trust me: do a little scouting now, and you'll save yourself a ton of stress down the road.

Get Your Blood Work Done

Ignorance is not bliss! Knowing your numbers will ease the concerns of curious parties (and contribute to your own peace of mind). It's a simple blood draw to test your levels of various necessary nutrients, and insurance should cover the bulk of the cost. At minimum, your panel should include a test of B_{12}, iron, and vitamin D status. Discuss all your testing options with a doctor or naturopath.

If your levels are normal you can flaunt them with confidence. If they're on the low side that's okay too - now you know where you'll need to put extra attention. Either way, it's much better to be informed than to remain in the dark. Knowledge is power and in my experience, being able to say *"Nope, not worried! I've been tested and my blood is beautiful,"* was priceless when facing skeptics.

Take A Picture
Your body is about to start morphing in a major way. So take a baseline body picture to reference in the coming months. Put on something skimpy and play supermodel! As your pregnancy unfolds, try to take regular photos of your changing form (I did it the first Wednesday of every month). Lining them all up ten months later offers some incredible visual impact!

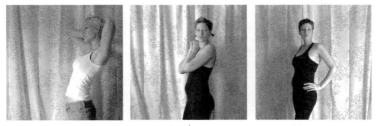

1 day   **12 weeks**   **16 weeks**

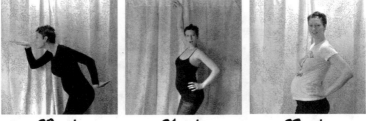

20 weeks   **24 weeks**   **28 weeks**

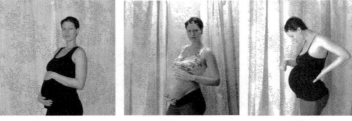

32 weeks   **36 weeks**   **259 days**

CHAPTER 2

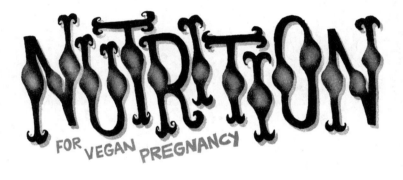

NUTRITION
FOR VEGAN PREGNANCY

Darling, you're building a person! There's no person there…and then, **there's going to be a person there.** That will never cease to blow my mind.

Of course, in order to make this magnificent human, your dietary requirements will change. This is true of carnists as much as it is of plant-eaters. Please rest assured: a vegan meal plan provides the full spectrum of nutrients that you'll need to assemble your brand new being.[8] Your job is simply to ensure that you're getting enough of those nutrients - *just the same as every other pregnant woman out there.*

D-D-D-Disclaimer - Did I mention that *I AM NOT A DIETITIAN?* It's true. I'm just some girl with a passion for health and a serious Internet addiction. The info I'm presenting here is pretty standard stuff, and it comes with the endorsement of our resident RD (he went to school for a *really* long time). However, I must disclaimer myself and direct you to seek your own professional assistance. Fair enough?

Nutritional Overview: The Big Picture

Pregnancy is a carousel of constant changes - hormonal, anatomical…and emotional. But amidst that madness, there are important things that you can control. You've got forty weeks to crank out a fully functional life form. This baby is baked from scratch, and you can make sure you're using the best ingredients available.

Let's talk energetics. Your calorie needs will increase by 10-20%, depending on the trimester. This is not the time to be restrictive! In the first three months you can expect to eat about 100 extra calories each day. Morning sickness may taunt your tummy, but do your best to keep the food coming. Your energy needs will rise again during the second and third trimester, when you'll be taking in 300-500 calories above your pre-baby baseline. But remember: this means 300 calories of kale, not 300 cookie calories![9] Make your calories count.

It's important to gain the right amount of weight[10][11]…but it's also important not to get stressed out about it. Experts suggest that the "normal" gain range is as follows: 25-35 lbs for women beginning with an average BMI; 28-40 lbs for women who are underweight; 15-25 lbs for those who start off heavy. But really, these are just guidelines. Every woman is different and every body will manage its pregnancy differently. You are unique, so discuss your specific weight gain goals and progress with your own prenatal provider.

As long as you're meeting your energy needs with *wholesome* and *varied* foods, you'll be able to build a beautiful baby. Contrary to urban legend, studies show that well-fed vegan mothers do not have smaller offspring.[12][13] In fact, a vegan diet may act as a preventative measure against common complications like preeclampsia.[14] So don't doubt your diet, okay? Go forth, and proudly eat plants!

"So, Like, How Do You Get Your Protein?"

You've heard it before but brace yourself: the bump brings on a whole new booming chorus of *"Where do you get your protein??!"* (My answer, by the way, is a big smile and a simple *"Plants!"*)

Now let's get something straight - as a general rule Americans are wholly over-proteinated. We tend to get more than enough and it's probably doing us more harm than good.[15] So don't stock up on Clif Bars just yet. You'll want to aim for upwards of 65-70 grams of protein per day[16], which is easily achieved without resorting to creepy processed products.

Pregnancy can make some vegans "protein paranoid", overcompensating with super supplements and strange meat replacements. But it's best to cull your protein from a wide variety of real foods, like legumes (beans, lentils, peas), whole grains (choose brown instead of white for things like rice and bread), nuts (all of them) and seeds (pumpkin, sesame, hemp, and sunflower are especially nutritious). Also remember that *all* foods contain the amino acids that make up protein. When you factor in fruits and vegetables, it adds up fast.

Let's take a moment to talk about quality. There's an old and unfortunate myth that says you need to invest your time and energy into carefully combining plants in order to create "whole" proteins at every meal. This is simply untrue.[17] ***You do not need to worry about combining proteins.*** Just eat a variety of protein-rich foods throughout the day, and your body will do the rest. Easy peasy. (And easy beans-y. And easy nuts-y. You get the picture…)

However, you're pregnant and playing it safe, and that's understandable. If you want to make sure your bases are covered, here's a list of plants that provide adequate levels of all nine essential amino acids:

amaranth – buckwheat – chia seeds – chlorella (green algae) – flax seeds – hemp seeds – nutritional yeast – oats – quinoa – soy – spirulina (blue-green algae)

Some of these foods may seem strange or exotic, but they're easily incorporated into an everyday diet. If you can't find them locally (check your health food store), you can get them all online. Try chlorella or spirulina added to a fruit smoothie, or hidden in a flavorful sauce (warning: start small because a little goes a long way, and know that they *will* turn your food bright green…which I think is fun!). Chia, flax, and hemp seeds can be blended into smoothies, sprinkled over salads, stirred into sauces or cereals, and tossed into breads or muffins. Flax is a baker's secret weapon: 1 tbsp fine-ground flax meal plus 3 tbsp water is a perfect egg replacer. Hemp is sold as seeds (the whole food), as milk (a great alternative to soy), and as protein powder (look for raw versions). Buckwheat is a pseudograin, often served hot as a breakfast cereal, called kasha.

It can also be ground into flour and used for pasta, bread, or other baked goods (buckwheat pancakes are amazing). Amaranth and quinoa are pseudograins as well - use them anywhere (everywhere!) in place of rice. Nutritional yeast is radical stuff - see the following section on B_{12} for more information. Oats are easy as breakfast or in baking. Did you know that a cup of cooked oatmeal has about as much protein as a large egg?[18] Soy is widely available in about a billion forms, and we'll talk more about that later.

The bottom line: as long as you're meeting your calorie needs and including enough variety - that is to say, not subsisting on processed carbs alone - **you will get enough protein.** But in case you're curious, there are free websites that allow you to track your daily macro- and micro-nutrient intakes. These can be helpful for squashing fears as well as pinpointing problem areas. I've used both *www.sparkpeople.com* and *nutritiondata. self.com* with good results.

Not All Carbs Are Created Equal

I almost didn't include this section. Do you really need me to tell you that unprocessed whole grains like wild rice, quinoa, and millet, are great for you, while refined wheat products like sandwich breads, crackers, and cookies, are crap? Do I really need to say "Hey! Low-carb diets are not nutritionally appropriate for a vegan pregnancy!"? Should I emphasize the shortcomings of simple sugars, while quelling the accompanying fear of fruit? (natural fructose + fiber = groovy, okay?) Must I remind you that wasting your precious caloric allotment on nutrient-poor choices like chips and cakes, is a bad bad idea?

(While gently reassuring you that if crackers are the only thing you can hold down in your first trimester, don't worry - you'll be okay!)

Do I really need to say all that? Naw, didn't think so.

Fat Is Rad

You may have spent your whole life fearing it, but listen up mama: fat is your friend! Of course, just like with carbs, *not all fats are created equal.* Steer clear of deep fried foods, trans fats, and anything hydrogenated, as well as cheap vegetable oils like soy and corn. But please, embrace those healthy fats. They've been unfairly demonized and it's time we recognize their benefits, which include improved skin elasticity and moisture (fight stretch marks!), lubricated…ahem…digestion (fight the bloat!), and most importantly, increased absorption of essential fat-soluble vitamins (like A, D, E, and K). Fat is an important part of a well-planned pregnancy diet. So load up on the good stuff:

avocados – coconut – nuts – olives– seeds

These foods are delicious as well as nutritious, and they'll add richness and satiety to your meals.

Vitamin B_{12}

Of all the micronutrients that cause concern for vegans, B_{12} is the most controversial - and the most confusing. Just a cursory bit of sleuthing unveils a variety of advice, which is often contradictory. You'll hear everything from,

"Animal products are the only source of B_{12}, which proves that vegan diets are unnatural for humans,"

to,

"Humans make our own B_{12} in our intestines, so we don't need to get it from our food,"

and every possible opinion in between. You know what they say about opinions...

The amount of misinformation out there is frightening and frankly, does a disservice to the movement. So let's look to the facts to clear a few things up:

- Vitamin B_{12} is absolutely essential for maintaining metabolic functions and for building your baby. You need it!
- **All B_{12} is made by bacteria** - it is present in animal foods because bacteria live on or in these animals and their secretions. This means **everybody,** whether omni or veg, **gets their B_{12} from bacteria.**
- There are no naturally occurring *reliable* vegan sources of *sufficient* vitamin B_{12}.[19] PLEASE DO NOT BELIEVE THE CRAZY PEOPLE ON THE INTERNET. You cannot get *reliable, sufficient* B_{12} from: seaweed, algae, bakers yeast (bread yeasts), mushrooms, tempeh, fermented foods, bran, sprouts, greens, "organic produce", or "by just not washing your vegetables".
- We *do* have bacteria living in our guts (bless them!) and they *do* make B_{12}. BUT. And this is a big but here - they

live too far down the digestive tract for us to absorb it. They make it, and we just poop it right on out.[20]

- It's true that most adults store B_{12}, stockpiled from a lifetime of steady ingestion. But this doesn't mean you don't need an additional, external source. Firstly, everybody is different and everybody stores B_{12} differently. You may burn through your reserves quickly and without realizing it. Secondly, your baby doesn't have any at all. Recent studies show that your stored B_{12} is unavailable to your baby, and only dietary B_{12} is transferred to the fetus or into breastmilk.[21]

It's a good idea to have your B_{12} levels checked when you get pregnant. Your prenatal vitamin will contain the RDA (recommended dietary allowance) or more, but many vegans choose to add a specific supplement on top (I did, as did most of the mamas I talked to). As well, you can incorporate B_{12}-fortified foods into your meals. These include: fortified cereals, fortified omni subs (meats and dairies), and many (not all) nutritional yeasts.

☞ ☞ ☞ All About Nooch! ☜ ☜ ☜

Nutritional yeast, affectionately known as 'nooch' to those who love it, is one of those freaky foods that vegans just seem to adore. Technically, it's 'deactivated cultured yeast' - I know, YUM right? - but in application it's the magic that makes the most amazing spreads, sauces, dips, and dressings. The flavor reads as 'cheesy' or 'nutty'. Nooch is crazy high in protein (~8 grams in 2 tbsp) and the B vitamins, making it perfect for pregnancy. Many brands (but not all, so check) are also fortified with that ever-elusive B$_{12}$. So give it a try. You may not love it at first - I've heard it's an acquired taste. But so is beer, and Tom Waits. Some tastes are just really, really worth acquiring. Dig?

👍 👍 👍 👍 👍 👍 👍 👍

For an exhaustive analysis of B$_{12}$ as it pertains to vegans, please read this review of the literature by Jack Norris, RD: http://www.veganhealth.org/articles/vitaminb12

Calcium

We've all heard that calcium is crucial in pregnancy. It makes up bones and teeth, and also plays a critical role in many metabolic functions. The recommended 'Adequate Intake' during pregnancy is set at 1,000 mg/day. And truthfully, meeting this goal can get a bit tricky, depending on your diet. Remember that calcium absorption is facilitated by Vitamin D[22], so eat calcium-rich foods with vitamin D-fortified foods. Or, pop your D sup with your tofu scramble. Or, eat your greens in the sunshine! (Just kidding, it doesn't work like that - though I'm sure it would be a lovely way to spend an afternoon!)

There are a number of factors that contribute to calcium loss as well. Excess sodium and excess protein both leech calcium from the body.[23] Too much caffeine[24] and alcohol[25] can also affect calcium retention. Greens are a great source of calcium, but greens high in oxalic acid - spinach, beet greens, and swiss chard - should not be considered a calcium source because the mineral is bound by the compound.

There's a common meme among vegans that goes something like,

"Animal protein acidifies the body, and an acid environment leeches calcium from bones. And excess protein also leads to calcium excretion. So, since vegans don't intake animal proteins and generally eat less protein overall, vegans don't need as much calcium".

This is a logical fallacy. Yes, there's some truth in there, but the scientific evidence does NOT support this conclusion. Period. Please don't believe that vegans need less calcium.

Your prenatal vitamin will include calcium, but only a fraction of what you need (between 15-40%). Thus you should aim to include 6-8 servings of calcium-rich foods each day. These include:

almonds – baked beans – black beans – blackstrap molasses – bok choy – broccoli – calcium-set tofu – chickpeas – collard greens – figs – fortified alt milks – fortified OJ – kale – mustard greens – navy beans, – okra – seaweeds – sesame seeds (unhulled only) and tahini (made from unhulled sesame seeds only) – tempeh – turnip greens

Here are some simple strategies for adding calcium to your diet:
- Stir a tablespoon of blackstrap molasses into your oatmeal. It may taste strong at first - start with a teaspoon and work your way up.
- Always choose tofu set with calcium sulfate, as opposed to nigari. This will be clearly labeled on the package. You can also check the calcium content on the nutrition fact

panel; calcium-set tofu will contain 20-30% DV per serving.

- Make up a trail mix of almonds and figs, and keep a stash in your purse. This is a well balanced protein/fat/carb snack that's great on the go - and very high in calcium!
- Hummus is a double whammy because it contains both chickpeas and tahini. However, note that most tahini is made from hulled sesame seeds, which contain a lot less calcium. Your best bet is to buy raw/unhulled sesame tahini, or to grind tahini from raw seeds, and make your own hummus. Maximize calcium intake by using it as dip for steamed broccoli and baby bok choi. Hummus can also be thinned with water and used as a dressing, served on a salad or over cooked greens. If you get bored of the standard chickpea hummus (blasphemy!), substitute calcium-rich navy beans or black beans instead. Both of these variations will make for a delicious dip.
- Learn to love your greens! They're great sautéed in olive oil and soy sauce, served with caramelized red onions. Or stir fried in sesame oil along with some tempeh or tofu. Or steamed with a pinch of salt and some nooch. Or, if you're crazy like me, try massaging some raw kale with avocado - it makes for an amazing salad.

If you'd like to learn more, the National Institute of Health provides a fairly comprehensive fact sheet on calcium, here: http://ods.od.nih.gov/factsheets/calcium/

Vitamin D

Oh, dear D, the vitamin du jour of our generation. You've probably heard all about this 'wunder-vite', as results roll in from a flurry of recent research. We now understand that vitamin D is invaluable for calcium absorption (deficiency leads to rickets, especially in children) and is integral to the immune system. The RDA is a paltry 600 IU (international units). I'm not going to tell you what to do, but I'll happily confess that I took 1,200 IU in the summer of my pregnancy and 2,400 IU in the fall-winter.

Vitamin D can get a bit tricky for vegans, as it comes in two distinct forms. D2, called *ergo*calciferol, is derived from non-animal sources and is vegan. D3, called *chole*calciferol, comes exclusively from animals and is not vegan. A little pneumonic to tell them apart: "I am vegan, *ergo* I take D2".

Vitamin D is produced through radiation - either real or artificial sun light. D2 is formed when yeasts are irradiated. We can take D2 as supplements and it will be converted into the usable form (D3) in our bodies.[26] Some research suggests that taking D2 is roughly 60% as effective as directly taking D3.[27]

D3 is made by all animals, including ourselves when our skin is exposed to sunlight. Some authorities insist that we need to take vitamin D in this form, while others disagree. I was quite confident taking vegan D2 throughout my pregnancy. If you want a complete review of the literature on vitamin D, you can find one here: http://www.veganhealth.org/articles/bones#d2d3 Make an informed decision!

Vitamin D is now included in most prenatal vitamins. And many "vegan" foods are fortified with D2, such as alt meats and alt dairies. More recently, "regular" foods like cereal and OJ are getting dosed with D. But watch out - many companies use D3, and suddenly your orange juice isn't vegan! Always, always read labels, and remember: "I'm vegan, *ergo* I take D2".

Other sources of vitamin D include mushrooms (very minimally, do not use shrooms as your only source) and of course, the sun. Aim to get 15-30 minutes of un-blocked exposure each day, but remember that variables such as skin color, age, and location will all affect how much D you actually synthesize. It is not advised to use sunlight as your only source of vitamin D, especially during pregnancy.[28]

Folate

Folate plays a key role in very early fetal development, and it's the vitamin most commonly associated with pregnancy. The RDA is 400 mcg pre-pregnancy and 600 mcg while you're pregnant. Luckily, this is one area where vegans have the upper hand, as we tend to get a lot more folate than omnis.[29]

So relax a bit in this arena. Your prenatal vitamin, which you should start taking before you even try to get pregnant, will have a heavy dose. And the following foods will keep you well over the line:

asparagus – avocado – chickpeas – grapefruit – leafy greens – lentils – OJ/oranges – okra – pinto beans – spinach – sunflower seeds – whole wheat foods

Just switching your white flour products to whole wheat ones (breads, pastas, tortillas, crackers) will add a whole slew of health benefits, along with an increase in folate.

Iron

*"How could you **possibly** get enough iron without eating meat?!"*

Not to make light of a serious situation - and iron-deficiency anemia is a common issue in pregnancy - but it sure is crazy how some people freak about iron, right? Like, since iron does duty in our blood, then the only way to get it must be from... blood? Ick.

During pregnancy your blood volume will swell (along with the rest of you), which increases your need for red blood cells. This in turn raises your iron requirements. But, being pregnant also causes you to maximize iron absorption[30], *because women's bodies are straight up spectacular!* But still, it's important to watch your intake. Low iron stores are associated with both preterm delivery and low birth weight.[31][32]

The RDA for iron is doubled during pregnancy, to 30 mg/day. Not all prenatal vitamins include iron, so make sure that yours does. This is especially important from the second trimester on. Risk of iron deficiency increases as the pregnancy progresses and is common in the third trimester (this is true of both omnis and vegans). So make sure to eat lots of iron-rich foods, like:

black beans – blackstrap molasses – cashews – chickpeas
– dark green leafies – lentils – pinto beans – potatoes
(especially skins) – pumpkin seeds – quinoa – soy beans
– sunflower seeds

Here are some easy ways to maximize iron intake:
- Always eat iron with vitamin C (orange slices on your greens; bell pepper in your beans) to really increase absorption.
- Switch to cast iron cookware, which will up the iron content of anything prepared in it.

☞ ☞ ☞ Personal Anecdote ☜ ☜ ☜

Like so many other women, my iron stores took a dip during my third trimester. I simply added a tablespoon of blackstrap molasses to my morning routine (taken right off the spoon, you get used to it pretty quickly). This worked like a charm to bring me right back up, and I'd imagine it would work as a preventative measure as well. And as a further aside, I began letting my son "clean" my molasses spoon once he was 6 months old. He never developed the iron-deficiency so prevalent in toddlers. Just sayin'.

👍 👍 👍 👍 👍 👍 👍 👍

Zinc

Zinc is oft overlooked in the pregnancy equation, but I think it deserves a mention. Zinc is important for cell division and the building of DNA, it aids in enzyme activity, it's a key part of immune system functioning, and it acts in many other essential metabolic processes. But pregnant women (regardless of diet) rarely meet the requirement. The RDA for zinc is 15 mg/day during pregnancy.

Make sure your prenatal vitamin includes a good dose of zinc, because not all of them do. As well, try to include a variety of zinc-rich foods in your diet. Some of these are:

almonds – cashews – chickpeas – lentils – millet – miso – pumpkin seeds – sunflower seeds – soybeans (including tofu) – tahini – tempeh – wheat germ

Zinc becomes more bioavailable in sprouted, soaked, roasted, leavened, and cultured foods. This is because these processes break down the phytates that would otherwise bind to the mineral. So to maximize your zinc intake:

- Try sprouting some sunflower, broccoli, or alfalfa seeds. Raw sprouts are great on sandwiches or in salads.
- Always soak grains and legumes for at least 8 hours before you cook them. Cover the dry product with plenty of water and add a splash of 'acid' (lemon juice or vinegar). Cover and let soak for >8 hours, than prepare as normal.
- Try soaking raw nuts (like almonds or cashews) or seeds (like sunflower or pumpkin) overnight. Then enjoy them with your breakfast - blended into your smoothie (makes it creamy and adds protein), atop your hot or cold cereal (along with fruit to add flair, ooh la la), or simply solo (though they can be a bit waterlogged and bland; an acquired taste).
- Toast up a pan of nuts or seeds. You can simply 'dry roast' these in a skillet on the stove over medium-low

heat. But keep a close eye, because they burn ever-so-quickly. Then toss them over salads or soups, eat them on your oatmeal, or create homemade trail mixes to keep on hand for snacking!

- Choose yeasted breads made with whole grains, over unleavened breads or chips or crackers.
- Choose cultured foods: tempeh over tofu, miso over other soups, and fermented nut cheeses (oh, you crazy vegan!).

Unraveling Omega-3s

Omega-3s are *essential* fats, meaning our body needs them and can't make them. They are important for brain development, attention span, vision, mood stability, disease prevention, and more. Basically, they're a huge deal. And unfortunately many vegans don't get enough of them.[33]

There are three forms of omega-3s: alpha-linoleic acid (ALA), eicosapentaenoic acid (EPA) and docosahexaenoic acid (DHA). ALA is a short chain fatty acid, while EPA and DHA are both long chains. DHA is the most advantageous omega-3, and the one you need to focus on during pregnancy.

You know how everyone is always going on and on (and ON) about how healthy fish is and how awesome fish oil capsules are? Well, that's because of the DHA. And a lot of people mistakenly believe that vegans *can't* get DHA since we won't eat fish. But yeah, no. In the same way that we get our calcium just like cows get it (from green plants), we can get our DHA just like the fish get it - from green algae.

Now, you may have heard that vegans can get their omega-3s from certain sources like flax seeds, hemp, walnuts, etc. This is true, but the omega-3s in these plant foods are ALA (remember, that's the short chain version). The ALA must then be converted to DHA in order to be used, and it's possible that the conversion rate is very low, as little as 4%.[34]

During pregnancy and breastfeeding, plant sources of ALA omegas are probably insufficient. You really should secure a solid source of actual DHA. These are widely available in supplements made from algae. Look for one that has 200-400 mg of DHA. Check your health food store or order online. Seriously, this one's important.

The Case For Supplements

I'm not a nutritionist or an MD, but I'm gonna go ahead and insert my opinion here. I think that supplements are really, really important. I take a prenatal/multivitamin, B_{12}, D, and DHA. This isn't just a vegan thing either. *I believe that everybody should be supplementing!* Here's why you should sup:

> 1) The quality of our food is atrocious. That includes locally, organically grown produce, too. Compared to the stuff our parents and grandparents were eating, food nowadays has a fraction of the vitamins and minerals.[35]

> 2) It's not worth being neurotic. In order to get 100% of every nutrient that you need, every day, *and* to eat a varied diet?... well, that's a full time job, man! And it's really

hard to do without eating exorbitant amounts of calories, because food just isn't that nutrient dense (see #1).

3) Being unhealthy is bad activism. Seriously, be a shining vibrant representative for veganism. Stay healthy and make the movement look *good*.

Some people say that they want to be "natural", that if we need to supplement it means that veganism is somehow "wrong". And I get that, I'm as crunchy - er, "natural" - as they come (dude, I use cloth toilet paper). But to that I have to say: "Sure…so let's stop eating anything that comes out of a box or a can, discontinue bathing daily, nix on using toothpaste (and tooth brushing at all, really), no more doctors, no more computers, start walking 4-6 hours a day, always go shoeless, and on and on. Then we can have a conversation about "natural", dig?"

We live in a modern world and we enjoy its many modern marvels. This is a blessing that helps make us better vegans. Embrace it! And be good to yourself.

Oi, Soy
There's a saying in the health community: *"If you're not confused about nutrition, you haven't studied it long enough."*

Nowhere is this more clear than in the raging soy debate (debacle?). There are thousands of studies and most of them contradict each other, making it easy to cherry pick data in order to make a case. The problem, of course, is that there are so many factors that play a role in human health. So one researcher may study a group of people and reach a solid conclusion, while another researcher may study a different group and come up with exactly the opposite. There are just so many variables and it's difficult to account for them all.

In the case of soy, you've got the detractors citing "proof" of *increased* cancer risk, thyroid suppression, hormone disruption, death to your ovaries, and ohmigod your son will catch the gay. Proponents can hold up just as many studies (SOMETIMES THE SAME STUDIES, OI!) claiming *decreased* cancer risk, reduction in heart disease, easing of menopausal symptoms, development of supersonic superpowers, and every time you eat soy a fairy gets its wings.

So who's right? Well…who knows? The jury's still out on this one. And it's possible they're both right - in the same way that wheat does damage to Coeliacs, soy may be acting differently on people depending on their individual physiology.

It's true that certain cultures have been eating soy foods for centuries with no apparent ill effect. It should be noted that this soy is eaten in moderation and most often in fermented forms (traditional preparations include miso, tempeh, natto, and soy sauce). Tofu and soy milk are more processed forms, and even more refined are the protein isolates found in many omni subs (meats, cheeses, etc) and other products (breads, condiments, etc).

It's also true that soy has never been consumed in such high quantities and in such altered states - seriously, it's in everything from muffins to marinades to fast food hamburgers. Soy is everywhere and all those little bits add up. And keep in mind that pretty much *all* non-organic soy is genetically modified, the consequences of which are sorely understudied.

Can you be healthy and vegan and soy-free? Yes! Should you aim to be soy free? Only you can answer that. I can tell you that almost all of the pregnant vegans I talked to DID and DO eat soy during pregnancy and breastfeeding, and every single one of them has a perfectly healthy baby. I can also tell you that I try to limit my own soy consumption. I choose non-soy options whenever I can (so for example, I'll buy almond or hemp milk instead of soy milk, use coconut oil instead of margarine, etc). If it's a matter of choosing which kind of soy, I always go for fermented varieties (for example when dining out, I'll pick tempeh over tofu). By consistently making these little choices, I don't have to worry when there *isn't* an option - "the coffee shop only has soy creamer, oh well", or "the restaurant's only vegan dish is tofu - I'll take it!"

This is what works for me - my body and my comfort level. I encourage everyone to do your own research and to find what works for you. I'd point you towards some unbiased info but, well, I haven't found any. Keep that in mind, too.

Keeping It Simple
I enjoy a long, lovingly prepared home-cooked meal as much as anyone. But sometimes - especially pregnant times - you need

something quick and simple. It's not always easy to know what to choose, what's healthy and what will keep you full and fueled. So I interviewed dozens of vegan mamas, and these were their top 'grab-n-go' recommendations for keeping life running smoothly when they were pregnant:

Apples (better with nut butter)
Bananas (better with nut butter)
Bars (Lara and Luna come highly regarded)
Beans out of the can
Cold cereals (can also be eaten dry for an on-the-go snack)
Dips (hummus or guacamole or salsa or bean dip) with veggies/crackers/corn chips
Granola/Granola Bars
Non-dairy yogurt
Nut butter and jelly sandwiches
Smoothies

It's All Just A Matter Of Choices

A little overwhelmed? I know, learning about nutrition can leave you feeling frazzled. It's just such a huge responsibility, this business of sprouting a whole new somebody! But sweetie, stress is the last thing you need. So try to keep things in perspective, okay? *This isn't about being perfect.* It's not about never letting a grain of sugar pass your lips, or compulsively keeping a food diary to track nutrients. Please don't drive yourself crazy.

This is just about being mindful. About remembering that it's not just you anymore. So one day at a time, one meal at a time, just practice making the healthier choice. Skip bagel day and opt for whole grains. Sub a salad instead of the fries. Go with a piece of fruit for dessert.

You don't have to think about overhauling your entire diet all at once. Taking it little step by little step keeps it much more manageable. So just focus on the food choice that's right in front of you, and make *that one* matter.

CHAPTER 3

TROUBLESHOOTING YOUR TRIMESTERS

There are already a million manuals to take you through the next nine months, minute by micro-managed minute. So we'll leave that to them. Here, we'll touch on some of the common issues that may arise as your pregnancy progresses, and discuss strategies for coping with them in the context of your veganism. But first, let's look at your treatment options:

Conventional. Unless explicitly stated, it's pretty safe to assume that all over-the-counter formulas have, at some point in their history, been tested on animals. That's just the unfortunate standard. Whether or not they contain any actual animal ingredients will depend on the product in question. The Vegan Society keeps a running list of medicines that are free of animal and their derivatives, available here: http://www.vegansociety. com/lifestyle/health.aspx

Homeopathic. Surprisingly, almost all homeopathic remedies are non-vegan. They routinely use a base of milk sugar called lactose. The two major brands, Hylands and Boiron, both use lactose, as do most smaller and independent vendors. Just recently I have begun to see "milk-free" and even specifically labeled "vegan" homeopathic products popping up. So if you want to try homeopathy, check your local health food store or poke around online.

Herbal. Most people hear the word "herb" and assume it's exclusively plant-based. Not so. I remember the first time I raided the storage room at my father's Chinese Medicine clinic. I pulled out a drawer and discovered a huge, whole dried seahorse. Trauma! Many herbal remedies, especially in Eastern medicines, are very, very *not* vegan. So be aware. And also be wary of the manufacturing country. Given their track record over the last few years, I tend to be distrustful of anything coming out of China. Lastly, please read the fine print. Many people I talk to are surprised when they go home and, upon my advice, examine the labels on their herb bottles…only to find a lead warning. That's right, lead. Not something you want to be ingesting during pregnancy. Keep an eye out.

And that's the situation as it stands. How you proceed in managing your own comfort is entirely up to you. You're a savvy lady, so trust your instincts.

Bloating & Gas

Bloating SUCKS. As one of the first indicators of pregnancy, bloating results from a spike in progesterone. I remember how I just couldn't wait to be pregnant, and also, how I couldn't wait to *look* pregnant. But 6 weeks in and suddenly I was blown up like a damn balloon. Not cute. And there's a lot of burping and farting, too. Woo-hoo! Bloating is just sort of one of those side effects you have to deal with during pregnancy, but there *are* a few things you can do to ease your discomfort:

- Drink plenty of water. Staying hydrated will help prevent constipation and keep everything - including air - moving along.
- Eat smaller amounts, eat slowly, and eat more often. Overfilling your stomach will stress your digestion. As well, when you eat quickly you swallow more air, which is a fast track to gas land.
- Move after meals. Take a walk, do a few sun salutations, whatever it takes to keep things in motion.
- Avoid your gas triggers, which will be different for everybody. Beans? Broccoli? You know your body, so listen to it!

Gas-X® is an over the counter medication that can offer relief from gas and bloating. Gas-X® Softgels and Prevention® both contain gelatin and are not suitable for vegans. But the Gas-X® Thin Strips® and Infant Drops are not made with any animal-derived ingredients. The company could not verify the status of the Gas-X® Chewables. All of the MYLANTA® gas relief products contain animal-derived ingredients.

If you suspect that food is the issue then you may want to try enzymes. Beano contains gelatin, but the brand Bean-zyme is a vegan alternative. The following herbs, brewed as tea, are also known for relieving gas pain: anise, chamomile, fennel, ginger, lemon balm, and peppermint.

Constipation & Hemorrhoids
Constipation is very common in pregnancy, when your hormones are all out of whack and your insides are squishing all over the place. The first line of defense against constipation is

hydration. Try carrying a refillable water bottle (stainless steel is best, but a glass mason jar is cheap and works in a pinch) with you at all times. A little lemon or cucumber slice can make it more appealing. It may help to set a cell phone alarm to go off every half hour, reminding you to take a sip.

The conventional wisdom for constipation calls for an increase in fiber. And that certainly works for some people. Me? Not so much. I eat a ton of fiber (like, a *ton*) and I lived with chronic constipation (hooray, too much information!) until I discovered two things: eating probiotic foods and consuming high doses of healthy fats. Probiotic pills and foods are excellent digestive aids. They keep your belly healthy and humming along strong. And along with daily probiotics, it's coconut oil, avocados, and nuts that keep me regular. So if you've tried the water and you've tried the fiber and you're still all backed up, why not branch out a bit? It may just blow your mind...and your bum.

Hemorrhoids usually pop up after too much straining to poop. If it ain't coming, quit pushing! The best thing you can do for hemorrhoids is to treat your digestive issues. In the meantime, a 'sitz bath' - a shallow, warm water soak - may help relieve symptoms (see *Herbs For Healing* in chapter 6). Most over-the-counter creams, such as Preparation H®, are not vegan. But the brand Earth Mama Angel Baby makes a wonderful "Earth Mama Bottom Balm" (not to be confused with the "Angel Baby Bottom Balm", which is great for diaper rash) that's all natural and completely cruelty-free. It's magical stuff...not that I would know or anything.

Edema & Swelling

It's normal to retain extra fluid during pregnancy, though "normal" does not equal "comfortable". Between the extra water, the slowed circulation, and the pressure on your veins, you might also experience swelling in your tissues - and that's edema.

The standard swelling from water retention may occur through the first and second trimester, while actual edema usually shows up in the final stretch. There are a few things you can do to help combat it:

- It may seem counter intuitive, but to retain less water you need to drink more water. You'll see this is a theme throughout this chapter. Water water water!
- Eat less salt and processed foods, as the sodium is a surefire ticket to Bloatsville.
- Move! Another common theme. If you sit for work, get up and do a little jig every half hour or so. Exercise as often as you can. Sedentary equals swelling.
- Uncross your legs. Uncross your ankles. Prop your feet up.

If you ever experience sudden or extreme swelling, or if your face begins to swell, please call your provider immediately. This may indicate the early stages of preeclampsia, which is a very serious pregnancy-induced condition.

Energy

One of the hardest parts about pregnancy is the damn fatigue. I remember thinking *"I have all this stuff to prepare for!"*, but being too exhausted to do anything other than surf a couch cushion. It drove me crazy!

Getting tired is par for the pregnancy course, but here are a few things to help you stave off the sleepies:

- Water keeps you alert and running in tip top shape - and at full speed.
- Go with the flow. If you really need a nap, then by all means take one. But set your alarm so you don't sleep all afternoon. Try giving yourself a half an hour to recharge. And of course, do everything you can to make sure you're getting enough sleep each night.
- Exercise. Walk around the neighborhood, visit the community pool, or get thee to a prenatal yoga class. If you have to, just do low-impact stretches in front of the TV each night. However you get it, regular exercise will keep your metabolism up.
- Stabilize your blood sugar. If you're relying too heavily on carbohydrates - even whole grains - you may be spiking and dropping your insulin levels. This is a huge tax on your system. Make sure you include enough protein and fat in each meal, and especially in your snacks. Between-meal eating tends more towards the sugary persuasion. Try raw nuts instead of dried fruit. Add hummus to your carrots or crackers. A handful of box cereal? Not great. A cup of oatmeal with pb and alt milk? Better. A small bowl of white beans with nooch? Now you're talking!

Food Aversions, AKA "Welcome to your first trimester!"

Everyone always harps on the cravings (they make for good comedy fodder), but most women find it's the aversions that hit first – and they come fast and furious. And since vegans tend to be passionate eaters, it can be pretty tragic when all of a sudden our favorite meals leave us heaving. Who knows why it happens? (certainly not scientists) What we do know, is that it's super sad.

The best technique is to make yourself adaptable. If the dinner you'd planned makes your stomach flip - well fine - you can move right along. Just remember to be mindful with your replacement meal. You shouldn't routinely be trading quinoa pilaf for a bowl of tater tots, okay? But as long as it's nutritious, it doesn't matter so much what you're eating. So keep an open mind, branch out, and allow yourself to sample some things you wouldn't normally choose. Who knows? You just may find a new food love.

Food Cravings, AKA "Welcome to your second trimester!"

Oh, cravings, the ultimate cliché. Sometimes they can be so delightful - for example, the sheer ecstasy borne of finally biting that long-desired fresh tomato and basil sandwich. Other times they're such a curse. Like when you're vegan, and 27 weeks pregnant, and pining for pork chops like mom used to make!

It's perfectly normal to crave strange foods during pregnancy, and many vegans find themselves lusting after animal products. You'll probably have people tell you that this is some sort of "sign". Like your body just *needs* to eat eggs/milk/fish/a double bacon cheeseburger. But the truth is that cravings occur for all sorts of reasons.

These strange and unexplained desires may range from benign infatuations with ketchup, olives, or ice, for example, to bizarre compulsions for dirt or detergent. The drive to dine on inedible objects is actually a medical disorder known as *pica*, and needs to be evaluated by a physician. And although your desire for burgers and wings may not be on par with a craving for clay, you can at least take heart in knowing that you're not alone in your struggle.

Food is celebratory, connective, nostalgic, comforting - all of the feelings that pregnancy invokes. There is no doubt that food is psychologically powerful. But our bodies are capable of misdirecting us; anybody who's ever smoked will tell you that. Just observe the obesity epidemic, alcohol addiction, and the success of Hershey's Chocolates as proof positive that our bodies don't always ask for what is in our best interest. Our cravings during pregnancy require that we intervene with our minds to assess the true needs of our bodies. And in most cases, it's an emotion that's actually doing the talking.

So please, don't cave to the cravings just because you think there's something you're not getting. The only thing you're probably missing is an old familiar flavor. Find a fabulous veganized version instead, or do something fun to distract yourself. But put your worries away - you're perfectly normal and plenty nourished.

Gestational Diabetes

Unlike aches, pains, and general fatigue, gestational diabetes is a serious affliction that needs to be monitored under the supervision of your health care provider. However, this disorder is intimately tied to diet, so I wanted to deal with it at least briefly.

I spoke with multiple women who were able to maintain their veganism while managing their gestational diabetes. *I want to stress that a lower-carbohydrate vegan meal plan is entirely possible.* GD can often be kept in check with menu modifications alone, and without the need for medication. This is true even with a more typically carb-heavy vegan diet. Please discuss your options with your doctor *and* a veg-friendly dietician.

Headaches

Like so many other pain-in-the-ass ailments, headaches are often a part of pregnancy. And like most of these afflictions, there's not a whole lot you can do on top of getting enough water and getting enough rest. Dehydration often manifests as headaches, so *do* make sure you stay plenty hydrated. If you need relief in the form of meds, there are tons of over-the-counter choices. Just watch out for these sneaky animal-derived ingredients: gelatin/anything in a 'gel cap', lactose, and pepsin. As well, the following ingredients may or may not have come from animals: glycerin, lecithin, magnesium stearate, stearic acid, and stearyl alcohol. It is generally recommended that pregnant women do not take aspirin.

Heartburn/Reflux

Pregnancy tests should come with a package of TUMS - which, by the way, are vegan!

Nothing ruins a perfectly pleasant meal faster than a bile burp. Ew. Here's a few time-tested tips for keeping heartburn at bay:

- Keep portions in check. If you fill too full you risk running over - right back up! Instead of three large meals, eat 5-6 medium ones.
- Keep trigger foods in check. Buh-bye to spicy, acidic, or fried. So sad, I know, but you've got plenty of other delicious alternatives.
- Speaking of eating, cut the midnight snack. Filling up before lying down is just asking for trouble. Abstain for at least three hours before you hit the sack.
- Speaking of bed time, try to sleep semi-reclined, with your head and shoulders raised. You can use a bunch of pillows to prop yourself up. This may take some getting used to, but it's well worth it.

There are a couple of different options if you want to treat your heartburn. The following antacids **do not** contain animal ingredients, though they come from companies that test on animals. TUMS (with the exception of the E-X Sugar Free and the Smoothies™ varieties), Alka-Seltzer Gold (avoid the original during pregnancy because it has aspirin,), and the following varieties of Maalox® Advanced: Regular Strength Liquid in "mint", Maximum Strength Liquid in "mint", "cherry", and "wild berry", and Maximum Strength Chewable in "assorted fruit" and "wild berry". Some women also swear by papaya enzymes/extract. These are now available at Trader Joe's (vegan and cheap!) and at health food stores (vegan-ness varies). Earth Mama Angel Baby is an all-natural, all-vegan company and their Heartburn Tea is reputed to work wonders.

Or, you can skip all that store bought stuff and just go DIY. Drop about a half teaspoon of baking soda into a half-filled glass of water (about 4 oz), stir until dissolved, and drink up. This is what I used throughout my pregnancy and it worked like magic. Oh, how I love baking soda!

Morning Sickness
Hooray, you're pregnant! You did it! It's happening! You've never been happier! Aaaaaand, then you get sick.

And so it goes, an upset stomach arrives early on to knock you down off your knocked-up high. Nobody knows why it happens exactly, and maybe you heard a rumor that vegans don't get morning sickness? Sorry, not true. Over 50% of women get sick, and that includes vegans.

So here, my dear herbivore, are a few guidelines for dealing with the queasies:
- Eat something the second you wake up, before you even get out of bed, and preferably something odorless and absorbent (like a cracker).
- Eat lightly, and try for "monomeals" (one food at a time). Especially avoid mixing fruit or fat with other foods.
- Eat often, as an empty stomach or low blood sugar can

quickly trigger nausea. This was my greatest weapon in my war on wooziness.

- Listen to your gut. It doesn't matter how healthy a food is or how much you used to love it. If it smells wrong or looks wrong, *don't force it!*
- Avoid strong smells, like perfumes and cleansers.
- Ginger and peppermint are both tummy tamers, so why not try making tea? Also, some women swear by the smell of fresh lemons.
- There are acupressure points in the center of the underside of your wrists. Stimulate them manually or pick up some Sea-Bands.
- Some studies suggest that supplementing with vitamin B6 is an effective treatment for morning sickness.[36] You can add a tablet or try these B6-rich foods: bananas, bell peppers, cauliflower, garlic, spinach, and most other greens.
- Take care of you. Clear out your stressors. Get a lot of sleep. Nurture yourself.
- Ultimately, don't freak out about what you're not eating. I promise that it will be okay. Before I got pregnant I had drafted up these elaborate meal ideas, like power smoothies and mineral-packed porridge. I was so prepared to load up on nutrients…but then I got sick and all I could eat for a whole month was popcorn. Sometimes you just gotta do what you gotta do.

Stretch Marks

Despite what the potion peddlers may tell you, all evidence indicates that stretch marks are mostly a matter of genetics. If you've gotten them before (from weight fluctuation or puberty), you'll most likely get them again. However, there are a few precautions that may be able to minimize the marks:

- Dry skin will crack, so keep your skin moist and malleable by staying hydrated. Yes, water is still a magical elixir of cure-all awesomeness.
- Eat your good fats, which will also keep your skin supple. Omegas are your friend.
- Apply healthy fats to your skin as well. Olive oil, coconut oil, jojoba, cocoa butter and shea butter are all great choices. Skip the perfumed and processed products.
- Avoid scratching. Your skin may itch from all that stretching, but fight the urge to scratch it. Itching probably means it's dry, so apply that oil and *rub* the tickle out.

Ultimately, stretch marks are what they are: a badge of birthing. So try to view them that way. Embrace them. They're your latest body mod, as beautiful as your last tattoo. Think of them as your tiger stripes and ROAR your way into motherhood!

CHAPTER 4

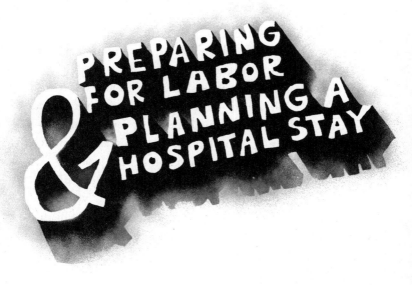

PREPARING
FOR LABOR
& PLANNING A
HOSPITAL STAY

The days are flying by and you've got so much to do. As you prep your workplace for maternity leave, you're also cataloguing a closet full of baby clothes, searching for the perfect pediatrician, and painting nursery furniture - all while Hypnobirthing mantras stream through your iPod ear buds. Mama, you are in overdrive! But try to take these last few weeks to really cherish the experience. Find a quiet place and sing lullabies to your belly. Take yourself out to get your hair done; splurge and add a manicure. Bake yourself something special.

If you have a partner, make sure that you're getting all the quality time you can. This is so important. You are about to embark on an amazing journey together, and it will be the most intense, most incredible, most difficult thing that you ever do with another human being. Now is the time to come together; to share your thoughts and your dreams and your sweet affection. Nothing will be the same once the stork makes the drop-off, so go on dates, hold hands, and give plenty of hugs. Just enjoy each other!

Okay, enough of the sappy stuff. You've got work to do mama. And as a vegan you'll need to do double diligence.

Feed The Freezer

Depending on where you live, it may be more or less difficult to get vegan convenience food. And believe me, convenience is exactly what you'll want once your baby joins the world. For this reason alone I can't rave enough about "feeding the freezer" - or in other words, making-big-ass-meals-and-freezing-them-in-individual-portions. I live in Portland, the "vegan Mecca", and even here it seemed like too much work to pick up take-out. Not to mention money! No, in the weeks following my son's birth, we pretty much lived off of the stockpile of soups I'd made and then frozen in my vast collection of mason jars. It was awesome.

So start saving jam and sauce jars. Clear out some space in your freezer. Then, fill it up. Some easy freezable meals include:

– chili – cookie dough (pre-rolled into balls) – curries (minus rice) – enchiladas – homemade granola/protein bars – "instant stir fry" of pre-cut veggies plus protein – lasagna – lentil loafs – muffins/sweet loafs – pasta sauces – pesto – pizza dough – pot pies – pre-rolled burritos – saucy casseroles – soups of all sorts – tamales – vegetable broth – veggie/bean burgers

Be Forward Thinking

This section is intended for those who are planning to birth in a hospital. But for all you home-birthers, it's not a bad idea to read through this too, in the unlikely case that you have to transfer.

There's plenty to keep you occupied during and after your labor, so the last thing you need is to worry about non-vegan items infiltrating your space. If you spend a little extra time now, it can save you a *lot* of extra effort in the future. Even those of you planning to birth at home would be prudent to do some hospital investigation. The chance of emergency transfer is slim, but it's always better to be prepared if you're going to be admitted.

- *Talk to your Docs* and make sure they're clear on what you believe in and why. Ask them to help you alert the rest of the staff during your stay. Remind them that veganism extends well beyond food, and reiterate that they'll need to discuss any medications or procedures before they proceed with them (this should be standard anyway, but it's a good idea to contextualize it within the veganism framework).

- *Call the hospital* ahead of time to make arrangements. Talk to the maternity ward and ask if you'll have access to a refrigerator, microwave, or other amenities (like a kettle or a cutting board). Then, ask to speak to the hospital kitchen and question them about your options. Many hospitals offer vegan meals...but many don't even know what vegan means. So scout out the situation to understand which one you'll be dealing with. Labor is hard work and usually leaves a lady starving - you don't want your first postpartum meal to be dry iceberg lettuce and soggy French fries.

- *Alert the nurses.* The nurses are your allies; they will interact with you far more than your primary provider. So buddy up and be nice! But understand, they have a lot to contend with and a lot of patients to keep straight. Make it easier on them by:

a. Writing a birth plan that includes a short explanation of veganism. Make multiple copies so that you can give one to each new nurse who comes on duty. Ask that one be attached to your chart.

b) Make signs to tape on your doors (at least 2 - one for the birth room and one for the recovery room). Something sweet and simple like, "We are vegan, which means we do not use any animal foods or animal-derived products. Thank you so much for the special consideration."

Bring Food For Labor

Many hospitals have policies that dictate what a woman is allowed to eat during labor. And this is important, because labor can go on for quite some time. A girl needs to keep her energy up.

The concern is that if by chance a cesarean section becomes necessary, the anesthesia may make it dangerous to have solid food in the stomach. In many hospitals laboring women are only allowed to consume "clears". This translates to jello, chicken broth, and an assortment of other very non-vegan items. So be prepared to bring your own labor "clears". Some excellent options (depending on the available amenities) include:

– coconut water – fruit juice – herbal tea – miso soup – popsicles – vegetable broth

If your hospital doesn't have a "clears" policy then you're free to eat whatever you want. Fruit, bars, and pb sammies all travel well. And don't forget to pack food for your labor partner.

Even if you've made prior arrangements with the kitchen, it's probably a good idea to bring along extra food for your stay...just in case. Focus on non-perishable, protein-rich foods (protein is the hardest vegan macronutrient to come by in an ill-equipped kitchen), like:

– a loaf of whole grain bread and a jar of peanut butter
– a number of those mini soymilk boxes so you don't need a fridge – energy bars like Lara or Luna – nooch and other spices to perk up pathetic veggies – trail mix with plenty of nuts and/or seeds – wasabi peas

Know Thy Meds
If it's possible you should talk to the staff ahead of time to learn about the hospital's post-partum protocol. For example, some medications are offered routinely, such as iron pills, multivitamins, and stool softeners. In many cases these contain animal ingredients or come in gel caps. As well, there are many drugs associated with labor itself - pitocin for example - that may not be vegan.

Whether or not you accept these or any other medication is entirely up to you. Remember that the definition of veganism, as stated by the Vegan Society (which coined the term), includes the passage -

*"...a philosophy and way of living which seeks to exclude - **as far as is possible and practical** - all forms of exploitation of, and cruelty to, animals for food, clothing or any other purpose..."*

This caveat, *"as far as is possible and practical"*, is an important one to remember in medical situations. Only you can make the call as to what constitutes "possible" or "practical" in your particular circumstance. But remember, that clause is there for a reason.

Also keep in mind that you can bring your own vegan versions of the pills they might prescribe, such as your prenatal vitamin or an iron tablet. For the constipation that commonly occurs post-partum, Milk of Magnesia may be a viable vegan alternative. Discuss this possibility with your provider *before you go into labor*, and be prepared to sneak everything past the nurses. I ended up smuggling an assortment of stuff into the hospital. I'd politely decline whatever they offered, then pop my own when they left the room. As long as we're just talking vitamins and their ilk, this should be fine and dandy. But please note, I'm not encouraging you to hide your use of pharmacological/psychoactive drugs. Be wise!

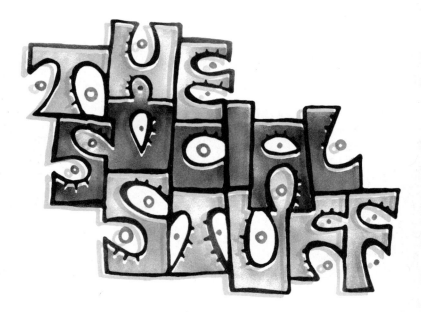

none of us live in a vegan bubble wonderland (no, not even in Portland). There are a number of common interpersonal issues that may arise throughout your pregnancy, and being prepared can help you to maneuver through these sticky situations.

Fielding Common Questions

In pregnancy there is no privacy, and everything personal becomes public. People will ask you questions that appear impolite. Some of these questions may be passive-aggressive critiques, but most will be borne of genuine curiosity or well-intentioned, however inappropriate, concern.

Think of these interactions as an opportunity for educational outreach. You get to be an ambassador of veganism, demonstrating health, confidence, and compassion. This is a chance to engage someone in a non-threatening way. It's truly one of the most effective forms of advocacy.

But, maybe you don't want to be the poster girl for a movement. If you're tired or "talked out", or just plain over it, it's also totally okay to plaster on the giant smile and say, *"I'm glad you're so interested in veganism! It really is a wonderful way to raise a child. I'll be happy to email you some more information. Please pass the dip. How about that weather?"*

If you do feel like engaging, here's a few of the most frequently asked questions, along with some ideas of how to deftly address them.

"Sooo, you aren't going to stay vegan, right?"
Sometimes a fib can carry you far. In this case, try a bit of feigned surprise - *"Why of course, why wouldn't I?"* - in your best Scarlett O'Hara *"Oh I do declare"* performance. Your bewildered response highlights how silly the question is. However, if they press you, be polite but clear. For example, *"It's just so easy to stay healthy by eating this way! There's less temptation and my food is naturally nutrient-rich."* By speaking of veganism with such confidence, you'll have them second-guessing why they were ever concerned in the first place.

"Did you tell your doctor that you're vegan?"
So much of people's doubt is rooted in fear. This questioner requires the permission...er...affirmation, of a person in a position of power. Allow them to defer to authority by assuring them that you've discussed it with your provider (which you should, but not because you need approval) and that you have their complete confidence.

"How do you get enough protein/calcium/iron?"
Here's where knowing your nutrition info will go a long way. Remember to remain calm and keep the quips in check. Bust-

ing out the knowledge will bring them around quicker than sarcasm ever could. Stay humble as you explain: Protein comes from legumes, whole grains, nuts, and seeds; we get calcium from green leafies and other plants, just as cows do; iron is in many foods such as dried fruit, nuts, beans, and greens.

"Don't you need to eat fish/take fish oil?"

This concerned individual is operating with incomplete info. They know that omega-3s (EPA/DHA) are important for fetal development, and they know that oily fish are the most common source of these essential fats. Now, it's just a matter of helping them to realize that there are safer and kinder alternatives. This is an important connection to make - that we can skip the middle man and get our nutrients from the same source as the animals themselves. In this case that's algae, which offers all the EPA/DHA goodness but with none of the mercury toxicity or environmental devastation. The abridged version: *"There's nothing in fish that I can't get from plants."*

"Breast milk is milk so it's not vegan, right?"

Other than blinking repeatedly with your mouth hanging open, here's how to address this one: *"I believe that cow's milk is for calves, and goat's milk is for kids. It seems to me a mother's milk, given freely from her very body to nourish her baby, is about as vegan as you can possibly get."* Some people may still miss the point - especially those who misunderstand the definition and purpose of veganism. Try putting it this way: *"Nursing a baby is AS vegan as the act of MAKING a baby. Both involve "using" an animal (sorry dudes!), and both are TOTALLY vegan. Kapish?"*

"What about that vegan family that starved their baby and it died?"

The unfortunate truth is that babies in developed countries still die from malnutrition all the time. This is an issue of parental neglect and it is always a tragedy. It's really sad that the media has irresponsibly sensationalized a few of these cases that involved vegans, because this is a serious problem that has nothing to do with veganism, and everything to do with negligence.

Here are a few other frequently asked questions, but the answers for these will vary from person to person. You might want to give them each some thought so that you'll be prepared to address them if they come up:

- *Are you going to breastfeed?* (Read: *"Is vegan breast milk safe/nutritionally adequate?"*)
- *Will you raise the baby vegan?* (Read: *"Is it safe/moral to raise a child vegan?"*, or, *"Don't you think you're depriving them of some sort of cultural experience?"*)
- *What if they want to eat meat some day?* (It's actually an important question for you to consider, but watch out - this person might be trying to play "catch the vegan".)

Handling Hostile Friends or Family

Sometimes, the people we love the very most can also be the biggest pain in our booty. And though our friends and family may have managed to keep themselves quiet about our "weird diet" in the past, they're much more likely to pipe up complaining once pregnancy is in the picture. It can be insulting, and infuriating, and when it comes down to it outright hurtful, to be challenged by our loved ones. But emotional reactions (however valid) are not necessarily prudent in the peace-keeping long run. After all, these are our nearest and dearest. We don't want to alienate ourselves and potentially deprive our babies of the familial love they deserve.

There's a few things that may help your case when dealing with less-than-understanding loved ones. First, call in the reinforcements. Make sure that your partner is in your corner and is willing to be vocal about it. It's harder to harass a "team" than it is to gang up on someone who's seemingly solo. You can also use the assurance of your prenatal provider to back you up. Make sure concerned parties know that your doctor approves of your lifestyle. And flaunt those test results!

Avoid emotional hot-topics like ethics and animal rights. That's an important conversation to have, but now is not the best time. Try to remain patient. Remember that these reactions are most likely coming from a place of genuine caring and concern. So channel your compassion. Calm down. And then, eat. Yup - E.A.T.

Education
Attitude
Take A Step Back

<u>Education.</u> Most people don't know a whole lot about health. I think you'll find that the majority of worry arises from a simple misunderstanding of basic human physiology. Therefore, if you can take the time to teach your comrades about

the ins and outs of vegan health, it can go a long way towards easing their fears. This is why it's so important to know your nutritional info. Study up on Chapter 2, and don't let anyone tell you that you can't get DHA without eating fishies! But when you correct them, try to do it ever-so-gently.

<u>Attitude.</u> It's the most important aspect of effective diplomacy. If you can radiate calm confidence, you'll be able to influence any audience. If you come off as defensive, unsure, or smug, you'll only hurt yourself. It's important to remember that it's not your job to change anybody's mind. Instead, you can only aim to explain the facts, to present your position, and to listen. If you can remain unattached to the outcome (like "converting" them), then you'll be able to keep your cool. Luckily there's plenty of science to back you up. So just stick to that - and SMILE.

<u>Take A Step Back.</u> Sometimes, even your sweetest, most Zen, most intellectual approach is met with anger and resistance. What can you do? If you've tried to be polite and you've tried to be brainy and you've done your very best being humble and sincere, well then, there's no shame in self-preservation. You've got much more pressing things to do than to worry yourself silly over somebody who won't play nice. At times like these, a little distance will go a long way. Remove yourself from the situation, not to be spiteful and not as punishment, but for your own emotional safety. Once you've had some space and are able to regain your composure, you'll have a better idea of how to proceed - either by attempting to come to an understanding, or by designating the topic as officially off limits.

There's a story that I keep hearing over and over again. Here's one version, as told to me by a woman named Cary:

"When my mother found out that I was going to remain vegan during my pregnancy, she was so upset. I would try to reassure her with my doctors reports that I was amazingly healthy. It wasn't until my mom came for a visit, ate the meals I cooked and met my little girl that she understood what veganism can do for a person. My mom and sisters are now also vegans."

A recent follow-up conversation with Cary revealed that not only is her conservative mother still a vocal advocate for veganism, but her big sister is currently in the midst of her own lovely vegan pregnancy.

So take a deep breath and be prepared to give it some time. You may have to wait a whole 10 months, but more likely than not your amazing, happy, healthy baby will go a long way towards building bridges. Best of luck!

Find An Outside Social Support Network
Not everybody lives in Portland, New York, or San Francisco. Midwest vegans, holla! Southern vegans, I hear ya! From the rural northeast to the arid southwest and in every teeny tiny town in between, there's a vegan representative. Y'all are awesome, and you have my respect.

It can be *so hard* to be the only vegan that you know. And pregnancy makes it even more isolating. But you don't have to go it alone! The Internet is a precious tool for forming community, so take full advantage. Talking to other pregnant and parenting vegans is invaluable and will do wonders for your wellbeing. Here are some ideas for using the Internet to find support:

- There is a website called Meetup.com that facilitates face-to-face gatherings for all manner of like-minded people. When you register you'll enter your city, and from there you can search for various local groups. Everything from Labrador Lovers to Pool Players to the Jonas Brothers Fan Club. Bigger cities have more specific groups - I belong to a *Vegan Families* group here in Portland. A smaller city may have a general *Vegans* group, and a town may only support a *Vegetarians* group. But poke around - you never know who's out there in your very own neighborhood.

- There are numerous active online forums specific to vegans. The websites www.vegtalk.org and vegpeople.com both have message boards designated for vegan families.

- There are hundreds of parenting websites out there, most of them pretty mainstream. If you're looking for something a little alternative, I recommend the forums at www.mothering.com. This is the community associated with the now defunct crunchy monthly, <u>Mothering Magazine</u>. There's a veg-friendly message board, as well as "Due Date Clubs" where you can virtually hang out with other mama's who are just exactly as pregnant as you are. I found it so reassuring to talk to like-minded women who were going through all the same stages as me, at the very same time.

- And finally, visit www.compassionatefamilies.com, the

companion website to this book. Hope to see you there!

Planning Parenthood With A Non-Vegan Partner

If Christians can marry Wiccans and libs can marry neo-cons, then surely a vegan can make it work with a mindful omnivore. In researching this book I spoke to many, many women who lived in mixed-food families. And though it may prove to be challenging, it's by no means impossible. Here are a few important pointers:

Talk About It Before You Get Pregnant.

This is one of those conversations that's better had with cool heads. Before you go mixing your genes up together, you need to be on the same page. Sit down and communicate. Gently suggest that your partner read up on the serious health affects associated with consuming animal protein. Be willing to ask yourself, what is important to you? (often this is ethics, animal rights, and/or health) And ask your partner, what is most important to them? (often along the lines of tradition, health, concern the child will be "different") Then, talk about how you two might reconcile your equally-valid-yet-opposing concerns. It might look something like…

Option A: The child remains vegan until they're old enough to decide for themselves how they'll eat/live. This will be different for every child, but usually falls somewhere between ages 7 and 10. Option A is appealing because it transfers the actual decision to the future child. Without the weight of what (and what not) to allow, both parties are able to relax…at least for the present. This choice also helps to remind you that this is a real person you're talking about here, an individual who will have unique thoughts and make their own self-interested decisions. That is super neat-o, so don't lose sight of the magic you two are about to make!

<u>Option B:</u> The child is raised vegetarian. This compromise may be a difficult one, as any vegan is well aware of the cruelty involved in milk and egg production. Still, you can certainly use vegetarianism to teach your child the values of kindness and compassion. Growing up without any meat will provide a solid foundation for transitioning to veganism later in life.

<u>Option C:</u> The child is vegan at home, but "omni when out". Another difficult compromise, but keep in mind that children do the vast majority of their eating at home. And you can insist on keeping an entirely vegan kitchen. But for the sake of your partner's stress levels, they won't have to worry about baked goods and hidden ingredients when they're out and about with the munchkin. The grandparents will be thrilled; you may have to do some mourning.

Make sure the conversation is appropriately framed.
The *choice* to eat meat is *as much* a decision as the choice not to eat meat, and if somebody says to you, *"You shouldn't force your own beliefs onto your child"*, then they clearly have not thought about their own inherent bias. Not to mention, what it is to be a parent! (By which I mean, I will certainly "force my beliefs"

that hitting is wrong, that stealing is immoral, and that gay people are equal, etc, onto my children. Because that's sort of exactly my job.)

But, don't box yourself in too tight.
With that said, the road will be less rocky if you can keep an open mind. As one animal activist shared, *"I was reevaluating **everything** from the perspective of a parent, of what life lessons I want to teach and what personal ideals I will not compromise, of the value I place on leading by example, and living and breathing the ideals that I want my child to know as truth."* In other words, it's okay to take a step back and reconsider what's important to you, and what you are willing to let go of.

Ideally, we'd all fall in love with people who see the world exactly as we do. Gosh, wouldn't that be swell? But life is messy and much more exciting. This is a conversation that needs to happen. Parenthood is hard - the hardest endeavor ever. Consider this good practice.

Planning A Vegan Baby Shower
It's your party and you'll veganize it if you want to!

It's surprising how often the issue comes up, from birthdays to weddings to family gatherings. And though you may have to make concessions when joining your family for Thanksgiving, your own baby shower is one time when you shouldn't have to compromise. I spoke with one woman who couldn't eat *a single thing* at her shower - even the salad had meat in it! - and she had to stave off a blood sugar crash with a bar she'd stashed in her purse. *Don't let this happen to you.* It is not unreasonable to request that your party be planned in accordance with your principals.

As always, stay respectful while standing strong. Don't let insensitive in-laws or a flighty friend hi-jack your celebration. Politely insist that nobody ever died from a few hours without animal products. A lot of omnivores simply have trouble visualizing a meal without the meat, so you may need to spend some time helping your party planners to see how many options they truly have. They'll worry about the guests but the truth is, if you don't make a fuss about it, most people probably won't even notice what's "missing".

If you're dealing with a veg-suspicious crowd, then the key for food is to offer up dishes that don't raise any red flags. Save the seitan roast for another occasion and stick to naturally vegan fare. If you're doing a serve-yourself spread you can't go wrong with Mediterranean mezza. Load up with hummus, baba ganoush, tabbouleh, tahini sauce, cracked olives, dolmas, and plenty of pita and crudités for dipping. Other buffet table favorites include chips with salsa and guacamole and bean dip, crackers with olive or red pepper tapenade, crusty baguette with bruschetta, and various cold concoctions like potato salad, pasta salad, and 3-bean salad. And of course, plenty of delicious fresh fruit.

If you plan to serve a sit-down meal, Italian is always an easy option. Everyone loves a killer marinara. Pasta primavera and pasta all'arrabbiata are also both naturally animal-free. But if pasta isn't your thing you could go in a number of different directions: creamy mushroom or asparagus risotto, vegetable skewers with tangy sauce, portobello mushroom paninis, Cuban black beans with cumin rice, pesto wraps, and the list goes on. Are you hungry yet!? Each of these pairs perfectly with a starter soup, a side salad, and a hunk of crusty bread, to round out a complete meal.

Clearly, there's an abundance of delicious and filling food options to keep your party-goers satisfied. But the other issue with showers is, of course, the gifts. Your friends and family may know that you're vegan, but many forget that this extends beyond diet. It can help to include a humble request along with the invitation, as baby gear is brimming with animal products: clothing made of wool, toys which may include bits of fur, feathers, and leather, care products that contain lanolin and bees wax, and books or toys with animal-exploitation imagery such as farms or circuses.

This can be such a delicate subject, and you may not be comfortable addressing it outright. That's understandable, and in this case a great solution is a registry. This way you can point people towards what you want. And know this: they will buy you gifts even if you tell them not to, so it's better that they have a list of acceptable items to choose from. Amazon is great because it's completely comprehensive and people can purchase and ship from anywhere.

You can also choose to buy everything that you need for yourself. This is the best option if you can afford it, because it allows you complete control. Of course, people are still going to want to give you gifts, and that's okay. Babies bring out the love in everyone. They'll want to express their caring through generosity, so let them. Be thankful. A great idea is to ask each person to bring their favorite childhood storybook. In this situation, you get a good head start on your baby's library, and your loved ones get to share a personal part of themselves. Everybody wins!

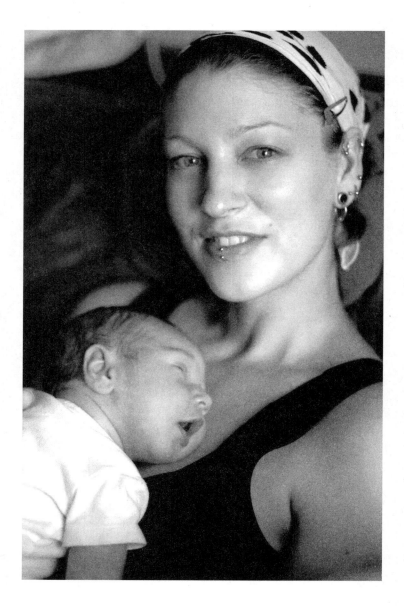

PART
TWO

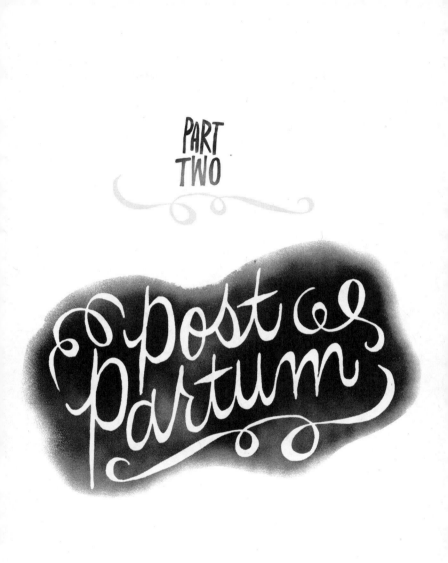

post
partum

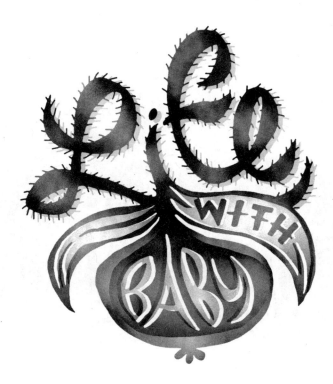

Hey mama, you did it. Bask in the gorgeous glow of new motherhood, and enjoy the bliss of your Babymoon. Yes, there will be diapers to figure out and a cord stump to clean and crying into the night. Oh, there will be meconium. There will, in fact, be all sorts of new and unexpected challenges ahead of you. And you'll face them - sometimes with grace and sometimes with humor and sometimes by the skin of your teeth - and you'll overcome them. Welcome to motherhood!

Introducing Pets

Animals are people too, and their reactions are as individual as they are. Some will assimilate immediately, quieting down and lying low. But others may feel jealous and vie for attention. Give them a little extra loving, but make sure they know to respect the baby. You wouldn't want them to see the wee one as competition. Conversely, some companions become "parents" themselves, welcoming the newborn as part of their pack. This sort of behavior is very sweet but must be monitored. Overprotective animals are prone to nipping at attackers...attackers like grandparents!

We're dog folks here, and our spoiled doggies sure didn't get it. At all. When we showed up with a mewling, strange-smelling bundle, they practically wriggled out of their skin with excitement. They had that crazy look in their eyes, the same one they get chasing squirrels at the park. It took a long time before they accepted our son as a human and not their newest squeaky toy. We had to be patient and careful, showing them the baby and softly cooing *"See, the baby, good boy, be gentle, no calm down, sit, good boy, see it's a baby, be nice, no licks, sit, good boy, be gentle with the baby, now calm down..."* and so on. It was weeks before we felt comfortable that they understood. But nowadays the boys are ever-patient as that tail-tasting, ear-tugging explorer tries again and again to climb Mt Canine. They're such good uncles.

Cats are a whole other ball of wax, as they tend towards independence and - dare I say it - indifference. Some kitties will be curious and you'll have to keep an eye out. Over-enthusiastic cats may want to get right up in baby's space, which is fine as long as you're there to make sure that Miss Thing behaves herself. Other felines may sense a shift in the mood and become mistrustful, hiding under beds or even refusing to come indoors. Do your best to make them feel welcomed, but don't force the issue. Cats are stubborn creatures and they'll come around when they're ready.

Mostly, your animals don't understand the implications of this monumental change. What they know is that their routine has been disrupted and there's suddenly a lot less attention aimed at them. So try to be sensitive towards their distress and even though you're surely stretched as it is, dig deep to find the time and emotional energy to give them a little something extra. Certainly, they deserve it.

Fore more great advice on acclimating your fur babies to your new baby, visit http://www.humanesociety.org/ and search for 'new baby'.

Placentophagy
Pla-what-in-the-whosit? You want me to WHAT?!
Oh yeah, I'm going there.

Placentophagy is a fancy term for eating the placenta. Yes, you read that right. Believe it or not it's a practice performed by almost every mammal, *including the herbivorous ones.* Though scientists aren't entirely sure why animals eat their afterbirth, it is known to contain three beneficial compounds. Firstly, prostaglandin stimulates the uterus to contract, which is a necessary part of post-partum recovery. Secondly, oxytocin is a relaxant and also plays a role in milk production. Finally, the placenta contains the Placental Opioid-Enhancing Factor, or POEF, that acts to decrease the pain felt immediately after birth.[37] Additionally, the placenta offers concentrated nutrients to the now-depleted mother. It's iron- and protein-rich with a slew of other goodies, meaning the placenta can help mama recoup what she has lost.

Many modern women have embraced placentophagy as well. The placenta is most often eaten raw, or cooked into a stew, or encapsulated into pills through a process of dehydration. The first two options are DIY; the latter usually employs a specialist. Very little research has been done in the realm of human placentophagy. However, there's a growing body of anecdotal evidence that's overwhelmingly positive. Advocates claim that the practice eases fatigue, balances hormones, promotes lactation, and most importantly, that it can help to alleviate or even prevent post-partum depression. Skeptics point out that there is no science to back up such claims. Which is true.

I ate my placenta and I'd do it again in a heartbeat. There's no doubt in my mind that it brightened my post-partum period immensely - both physically and emotionally. I froze it raw and hacked off a small sliver each morning to blend into my smoothie. It lasted me almost three months. Some may claim that what I experienced was the placebo affect, to which I counter *"Who cares!? It worked and it was awesome!"* I only wish I had a never-ending supply of that magical little membrane.

Foods To Fight The Baby Blues

It's very normal to feel an emotional drop in the days and weeks after giving birth. And why not? You went through a serious physical ordeal, you lost a lot of blood and tissues, and your hormones are all out of whack. Plus now your time is taxed, you're sleep deprived, and you've become a milk machine. All of it adds up, and how could it not affect you? But luckily, you can begin to manage your moods through your diet and lifestyle.

Ideally you've been taking an omega-3 supplement throughout your pregnancy, but if you haven't then you should start now.

There's a growing body of research that links higher levels of DHA to lower instances of depression.[38][39][40] DHA is also vital to your baby's growing brain[41], so this is especially important if you're breastfeeding. If you don't like the idea of taking a supplement, you can obtain the precursor omega-3s from flax, hemp, and walnuts. (See chapter 2 for more information.)

In general, it's a good idea to treat your body with extra kindness in these first few postpartum months. There may not be any science to prove it, but common sense says that nourishing, whole foods will leave you feeling worlds better than processed, out-of-a-box stuff. So load up on smoothies, salads, and other fresh, hydrating fruits and veggies. There's even some evidence that a higher-carb (*good* carbs) diet can help to combat postpartum mood swings.[42] Yay vegan!

There are also a few lifestyle choices that can keep you on track towards emotional stability. First, try exposing yourself to sunlight for at least 15 minutes every day. Aside from the vitamin D, the fresh air and the feeling of warmth on your skin will works wonders on your mental state. Conversely, avoid stimulants like caffeine and sugar. Especially sugar. Sugar wreaks havoc on your whole system and it's a one-way ticket to anxiety-town. Sorry friend. Try to steer clear of depressants, like alcohol and pot, as well. Hold off until you're sure that your emotions are under control. Certainly, it's true that a glass of wine and a hot bath can go a long way for a hardworking new mommy. But save the celebration until after your body has recalibrated. Then have at it mama - you'll deserve it!

Herbs For Healing (Mind and Body)

Giving birth is like a physiological tornado. Organs have been relocated, fluids have changed composition, your very bones have bent…and most likely some membranes have torn. Regardless of how your labor unfolded, there will be healing to do.

A lot of women, and especially new and breastfeeding mothers, are hesitant to use conventional curatives full of harsh chemicals. And of course, most over-the-counter concoctions aren't vegan anyways. Boo! But that's okay - the most common postpartum ailments can be addressed with homemade alternatives.

Many of these are best made prior to birth, to have on hand when the need arises. As a bonus, the preparation process itself is great for channeling nervous energy in the weeks leading up to labor. So why not cut two carrots with one knife? Keep yourself busy now and you'll keep yourself comfortable later.

<u>Healing Herbs</u>

Alfalfa: A very nutritive plant. Drink as a tea to replenish minerals and to energize. It's also believed to promote lactation. Do not use alfalfa if you have, or have a family history of, lupus.

Aloe Vera (fresh only): Squeeze the jelly from the leaves and dab it onto a tear/episiotomy. Allow to air dry after application.

Arnica: Use an infused oil on bruising/sore areas (perineum, vagina, even tired legs) but keep it out of open wounds. Can be irritating if over-used. Do not take arnica internally.

Blessed Thistle: Taken as a tea or infusion, it decreases uterine bleeding, stabilizes irritability and anxiety, facilitates digestion, and boosts milk production. The perfect postpartum herb? Methinks it may be!

Blisswort (aka Skullcap): An excellent sedative herb for restoring energy and calming nerves. Especially good for adrenal fatigue (common in new moms). Best taken as a tincture but tea works as well.

Calendula Flower: Use in a sitz bath for wound healing and hemorrhoids, or on a compress or postpartum pad to soothe tears and stitches. Anti-inflammatory and antimicrobial, it stimulates tissue development.

Chamomile: Both a stress reliever and a tummy tamer, chamomile is mom's best friend. Brew a blend of chamomile, catnip, and lavender for ultimate relaxation. Bonus! – this mixture will help to calm colic via breast milk.

Dandelion Leaf: Nourishing and high in trace minerals, drink as an infusion to rebuild your nutrient stores. The leaves can also be picked fresh (weed your yard!) and cooked like kale or other greens, or tossed into green smoothies. Dandelion promotes milk production and can also be used in a compress to ease mastitis.

Fennel: Eaten as seed or brewed into tea, fennel is great for digestion and increases milk supply.

Jasmine: Crushed flowers may be rubbed on the breast to stimulate milk flow. Make sure to wipe it clean before nursing.

Lavender: Add a diluted infusion in a peri bottle to soothe and keep clean after urinating. Use in a sitz bath. Take as a tea for calming or to increase milk supply. Analgesic (pain killer), antimicrobial, and antidepressant.

Nettle Leaf: A nutritive herb that's chock full of good stuff, drink it as a tea to fight fatigue and rebuild your mineral stores. Combats postpartum anemia and enhances breast milk. A real power player - highly recommended!

Oatstraw: Another nutritive herb, mineral-rich and replenishing. Brew in a strong infusion to drink as tea.

St. John's Wort: Use with other herbs in a sitz bath or on a compress for hemorrhoids or tearing.

Strawberry Leaf: Drink as tea before bed to stave off night sweats.

Witch Hazel: Use in a sitz bath or on a compress or postpartum pad to soothe hemorrhoids. Can also be used in an oil or on a compress to combat varicose veins. Anti-inflammatory, astringent (reduces swelling), and haemostatic (helps stop bleeding).

Infusions: An infusion is easily made by pouring boiling water over herbs and allowing the mixture to steep for an extended period - often overnight. A good general rule is 1/2-1 cup herbs to 4 cups water. Infusions can be taken internally or applied externally.

☞ ☞ Sayward's Restorative Postpartum Infusion ☜ ☜

Combine 2 parts nettle with 1 part each of alfalfa, dandelion, and oatstraw. Brew strong (1 cup herbs to 4 cups water) and steep overnight. Drink daily for…ever? I'm still drinking variations of this almost every evening (brewed with other teas for flavor and served over ice), and I have no plans of stopping.

👍👍👍👍👍👍👍👍

Compress: Premade witch hazel wipes can be purchased at many natural markets. You can also easily make your own, by soaking strips of cotton or cloth in an herbal infusion. Use these to soothe hemorrhoids, minor tears, bruising, and stitches.

Sitz: A healing sitz bath is made by adding a few tablespoons of herbs to a few cups of boiling water and allowing this to steep for 20 minutes. The resulting infusion is then added to a very shallow bath. Use a single herb like lavender, or combine several types like chamomile and calendula flower. You can add 2-3 drops of essential oil such as cypress, lavender or tea tree. You may also include sea salt or a fresh clove of garlic. Herbs to promote perineum healing include: burdock, calendula flower, ladies mantle, lavender, lemon balm, oak bark, rosemary leaf, St John's wort, witch hazel, and yarrow flower.

Pads: Postpartum pads are super rad because they soothe and heal all at the same time. Begin by purchasing some extra large, super absorbent maxi pads. Then make an infusion of calendula, lavender, witch hazel, or any combination of these. Lay the pads out on a baking tray, spoon the infusion onto them, and then place the tray in the freezer. Once the pads are frozen you can stack them for easier storage. Make a bunch of batches and wear them constantly in the days following the birth. The cold + herbs = bliss. Hallelujah.

Much of the subject matter outlined in this chapter is alternative in nature. Please discuss all your options with your doctor or midwife, especially if you experience depressive or destructive thoughts after giving birth.

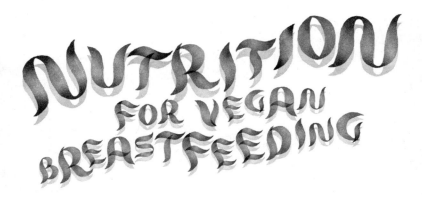

you didn't think you were done with nutrition, now did you? Consider this: during pregnancy you're given nine months to grow a baby from zero to eight-ish pounds (give or take a few). But over the first year of life, your baby will pack on an easy 12-18 more. That's roughly double the growth! Not to mention the brain development, motor skills, and eventual locomotion that demands so many calories along the way. The bottom line: being solely responsible for another creature's entire energy needs is a demanding job. Lucky for you, you're in good company. Vegans are much more likely to breastfeed, and to do so for closer to the 2 years recommended by the World Health Organization. Bonus: we also have significantly less toxins in our milk - less pollutants, pesticides, and PCBs. [43] Yay vegan!

Why Breastfeed?
Simply put, if you *can* do it then breastfeeding is the best thing for your baby. Period! It's also great for you, and for your way of life as well. Here's just a sampling of the many breastfeeding benefits[44]:

For Baby

- Much easier digestion (less gas, less constipation, and less diarrhea).
- Lowered chance of colic.
- Stronger immune system and acquisition of maternal immunities. This includes less instances of bacterial/viral infection such as meningitis.
- Fewer ear infections, all the way through childhood.
- Fewer allergies.
- Fewer instances of asthma, pneumonia, or other respiratory issues.
- Higher IQ and scholastic success, all the way through to the college level.
- Less likelihood of childhood obesity and diabetes.
- Lowered risk of cancer.
- Decreased instances of SIDS.
- Better dental development and fewer cavities.

For Mom

- Promotes important initial bonding.
- Causes uterine contractions that help to prevent postpartum bleeding.
- Aids postpartum weight loss.
- Delays menstruation (which helps retain iron, among other things).
- Decreases the chance of developing reproductive and breast cancers later in life.
- Promotes bone health and reduces the risk of osteoporosis.
- Reduces the chance of developing type II diabetes.

As A Lifestyle
- There's no prep work - no heating, no can opening, no bottle washing. Talk about convenient!
- Totally portable and always available.
- Saves hundreds if not thousands of dollars.
- Super quick - no time wasted prepping formula means that baby's needs are met immediately.
- No risk of food borne illness or water contamination.
- It's green! No shipping, no packaging.

Most importantly, breast milk is, quite literally, the perfect food for your baby. It comes complete with every necessary vitamin and mineral and in all the appropriate macronutrient ratios (that change throughout the day and also over time, to suit your babies needs - hello magic milk mother!) And yes, *it's totally vegan!!!*

Nutritional Overview: The Big Picture
As with baking your baby bun, creating a toddler requires a huge energetic input. During the first year of life your baby will develop faster than at any time in the future, and all of that energy - ALL of it - is coming from you. Little bones are built from the calcium you consume; baby brains flourish with the fatty acids found in your food, neurons and nails and every last eyelash, is made from mama. Now is the time to redouble your commitment to nourishing foods.

By the end of your pregnancy you were eating an extra 300 or so calories each day. Now, that number climbs as high as 500. For reals! But don't worry, unlike the last few weeks of pregnancy, you will definitely be hungry. (What, you didn't lose your appetite at the end of your pregnancy? Yeah, neither did I.) Keep in mind that vegan food tends to be nutrient-dense but calorie-light, so make sure that you have easy, healthy snacks available. Choose high-energy foods such as nuts/nut butters and seeds/seed butters, dried fruit, and healthy whole food-based fats like avocados and olives. Remember my rule: kale calories, not cookie calories!

You may be itching to shed that extra pregnancy weight, but now is NOT the time to diet. If you eat nutrient-dense foods and eat to satiety, you should experience slow and steady weight loss. *It will take a while.* For some women, breastfeed-ing causes the weight to melt away, and they're back to their svelte shape in no time. For other women, their bodies hold onto some "nursing pads", a few extra pounds that will stick around until their child weans. Whatever your body decides, try not to fight it as it works to feed your baby. Just focus on eating right and leave the body image anxiety for a few years down the line, when you're all done building new people. Or, you know, never.

Hydration And Hydrating Foods
Breastfeeding can be surprisingly drying. Milk is made with water, after all, and not drinking enough can cause your milk supply to drop. You may also notice rough skin, dry eyes, and chapped lips - all indications that you need to increase your fluid intake. It's very important for both you and your baby that you take extra care to stay hydrated.

Try keeping a canteen in your purse, your car, your diaper bag, and next to your nursing throne - err, I mean chair. Any and every time that you sit down to feed your baby, make sure that there's a tall glass of water nearby. You may not want it before you begin to nurse, but as soon as the little one latches on, The Thirst™ will come. Seriously, it's like clockwork! As always, a slice of lemon or a few raspberries can make boring water so much more appealing.

Other fun ways to expand your liquid repertoire include: coconut water (which is full of vitamins and minerals and electrolytes), green tea (no, the caffeine will not dehydrate you, but make sure your nursling doesn't react to it), herbal infusions (see chapter 7), juicy fruits like melons and citrus, and fresh raw veggies (especially cucumber, celery, and salad greens).

Don't Get Depleted!
Diet affects breast milk composition, but only to a certain degree. The truth is that if your nutrient intake is insufficient, then your milk-makers will simply steal from your own private stores. In other words, it's *you* who will probably suffer mama, not your baby. (The exceptions include omega-3 fatty acids, iodine, manganese, selenium, and vitamins B_9 (folate), B_{12}, D, and K. In these cases insufficient consumption may mean lowered levels in milk.)[45]

Most new moms of all dietary stripes find themselves feeling fatigued, foggy, and generally run-down. This is often caused by a killer combo of sleep deprivation, hormonal adjustment, and stress. But nutritional depletion can certainly add fuel to the fire. So make sure that you continue to take your prenatal vitamin and any other supplements that you may have used during pregnancy. As somebody with absolutely no official authority to make nutritional recommendations, I strongly suggest including B_{12}, D_2, and DHA on top of your prenatal.

Aside from supplements, there's quite a lot that you can do with your diet. Including the following 'mega-mineral' foods will help to ensure that you stay healthy and strong through what is often a tough postpartum period. These foods offer the ultimate in nutrient density, as well as providing a wide spectrum of key trace elements. Use them!

Cultured/Fermented Foods (like yogurt, sauerkraut, kombucha, etc) - Probiotics are essential to digestive health, and they allow you to maximize absorption from everything that you eat. Probiotics also aid immune function and can be passed to your baby. A healthy gut is the key to a healthy human - so eat your probiotics!

Here's How: Nondairy yogurt makes a great breakfast on it's own or added to smoothies. Sauerkraut or other fermented vegetables are lovely as an appetizer or simply as a side to accompany any meal. Kombucha and water kefir are delicious fizzy beverages and both are easy to make at home. All fermented foods are detoxifying, so breastfeeding moms need to start with small portions and slowly increase their intake over time.

Dark Leafy Greens (like chard, collards, kale, etc) - High in calcium, folate, iron, magnesium, potassium, and vitamins A, C, E, and K. These have tons of protein per calorie, as well as phytonutrients and antioxidants. They even contain essential fatty acids!

Here's How: The vitamins in greens are fat-soluble, so make sure to pair them with a good source of fat. If you can't tolerate their flavor, try them blended into a fruit smoothie (raw, starting small and working up as your taste acclimates). Otherwise enjoy them raw in salads (microgreens, arugula, or kale massaged with olive oil) or cooked into soups (shred them and stir them in right before serving), incorporated into stir frys, or on their own (sautéed in oil with garlic and ginger or with leeks and shallots).

Herbal Infusions (like alfalfa, dandelion, nettle, oatstraw, and red raspberry leaf, or a combination of any/all) - Nutrient composition will vary by plant, but includes the major minerals calcium, iron, phosphorous, potassium, and sulphur, as well as many trace minerals. These herbs are also high in vitamins A, C, E, and some of the Bs.

Here's How: For more information on nutrition and preparation, see chapter 6.

Lentils - Aside from their impressive protein load, lentils are exceptionally high in iron. They're considered a good source of folate, thiamine, and other B-vitamins. Lentils also contain copper, manganese, molybdenum (a mineral with many functions including dental health), phosphorous, and potassium.

Here's How: Lentils cook up easy compared to other legumes. You don't need to soak them (though sprouting increases their nutritional profile). Just bring them to a boil and simmer for 20-30 minutes. Spice and season and voila - healthy dinner! There's a billion recipes available all over the place. Dig in!

Blackstrap Molasses - This gummy black syrup actually contains up to 20% of the required daily calcium and iron, all in a single tablespoon. There's other trace minerals as well, but molasses are mainly used as a food-based iron/calcium supplement. Make sure you get blackstrap, as opposed to mild/barbados, dark, or sorghum syrup.

Here's How: I think the easiest way to include molasses is straight off the spoon. The first time I did it I gagged, but by the end of the week I was gulping it down and happily licking the leftover drops. A tablespoon a day corrected my third trimester anemia and has kept my breastfed baby from developing the oh-so-common low iron stores. He loves to clean my spoon!

If you can't handle the stuff straight up, try it in a smoothie (start with a teaspoon) or stirred into hot cereal. I always add a good glug to my lentil soups and other stews. But although it may sound appealing, the tiny amount of iron that you get from molasses cookies is not really worth the sugar trade-off. Sorry!

Fortified Nutritional Yeast - (make sure you buy a 'fortified' brand such as Red Star) Nooch is very high in protein and in the suite of B-vitamins, including B_{12}. Truly a vegan wonder-food - sprinkle it over popcorn, pasta, beans, salads, hummus, corn chips, or anything else your heart desires.

Here's How: See chapter 2 for more information on nutrition and preparation.

Green Pumpkin Seeds - One of the best plant sources of zinc, and high in the minerals copper, iron, manganese, magnesium, and phosphorous. They also provide protein, vitamin k, and omega-3 fatty acids.

Here's How: Pumpkin seeds can be an acquired taste and may be tricky to incorporate into meals. You can always eat them plain - a handful here or there - or as part of a trail mix. They're also good sprinkled atop stir frys, fresh salads, and hot or cold cereals. They're awesome in place of pine nuts to make a pesto! If you have a high-speed blender, you can also hide them in smoothies.

Sea Vegetables - Iodine is an incredibly important and often overlooked trace mineral, and sea veggies are a great way to ensure you're getting it. You need iodine to regulate your thyroid, which is especially vulnerable during and after pregnancy. Iodine is important! On top of this essential nutrient, most sea vegetables also provide a hefty dose of both iron and calcium.

Here's How: There are many types of sea veggies and they all taste unique, so you may want to experiment. Nori is the classic sushi "wrapper", great for homemade sushi but also for easy wraps. Hummus, nut butter spreads, seed pâtés, etc, all taste great wrapped up with veggies in a sheet of nori.

Wakame is a calcium-rich seaweed that usually comes in dried form. Rehydrate it in water and then toss it with sesame oil and lemon juice. Top with sesame seeds and avocado for a quick snack. Dulse is another popular variety that you'll find sold as small flakes. You can serve it in soups or salads, or mash it with chickpeas and vegan mayo for a tasty tuna substitute. There are tons of sea veggie choices, so make sure you explore your options!

Eating Well With No Time To Spare
Healthy eating is hard enough when it's just you and your own life to juggle. Add in your brand new role as mother with a brand new baby to care for, and the only recipe you'll be following is one for disaster! I kid, of course, and I promise you that disaster is not actually imminent (though I'm sure it will feel like that sometimes). The key is to make sure you're eating right when you're already stretched to paper thin and it would be so much easier to just zap a microwave meal.

Here's a few easy tips:
- First, stash that microwave in the garage/attic/basement/not-the-kitchen. Remove the temptation! Anything worth eating can be heated/re-heated on the stovetop.
- Late night or early morning prep will be your lifesaver. Use that precious time when the baby is sleeping soundly: if you're a morning person, just get up a little earlier. If you're a night person, putter in the kitchen

to unwind after a long day. Either way, put on a podcast or some soothing music and relish in some 'you' time, meditating as you chop stacks of carrot and celery sticks, clean and core bell peppers, slice up cukes, and dice up onion. Now is also an excellent time to make a few dips, which will keep for a week in the fridge. With hummus and pre-cut veggies on hand you won't have to reach for those cookies!

- Use your "weekend" kitchen time. Whether your "weekend" is Saturday and Sunday when your partner is home, or Tuesday afternoon when your mom drops by, take advantage of hands-free time when somebody else is holding the baby! In an hour you can construct a casserole, simmer a stew, and whip up a batch of whole grain waffles, all of which can be frozen in individual portions for easy access during the week.

- Calling Your Crock Pot! Dig that old thing out from the back of the cupboard (or get thee to the thrift store and pick one up on the cheap). Your crock pot is your best pal. A couple cups of beans, a couple more cups of water or broth, and by afternoon you've got a steaming pot of protein-y goodness. I make a crock of beans a week: some go into a soup that gets eaten a few nights and then frozen for later; others stay plain and sit in the fridge. They're awesome to have on hand for snacks or lunch. A bowl of beans plus nooch and spices is super easy, filling and delicious!

- I'm a huge advocate of smoothies, especially the green variety. But it's true that they can be a bit time consuming when you're just making one. However, you can make smoothies in big batches and save the rest for later! Fill your entire blender up and then bottle the excess in mason jars. They'll keep for up to 48 hours in the fridge, or indefinitely in the freezer.

• If your partner works long hours or your family lives far away or if you're a single mum hacking it on your own, you've still got one card up your sleeve: you can wear your baby in the kitchen! In a sling, a pouch, or a wrap, get your baby used to being worn around the house. This offers oh-so-necessary two-handed time when you're by yourself. Lots of little ones will learn to fall asleep while being worn, and you'll be free to cook and clean as you need. Practice makes perfect and remember to keep those toesies away from hot pots!

Vegan Galactagogues

A galactagogue is a really cool word that's hard to say. Oh! And it's also any substance that increases your milk supply. So if you're not making enough milk, try these natural booby boosters (please consult with a lactation counselor first; Le Leche League is free and wonderful, call 1-800-LALECHE). The best herbal and food-based galactagogues are as follows:

Alfalfa
Anise
Asparagus
Blessed Thistle
Brewer's Yeast
Fennel
Fenugreek

Flax
Hops (including beer, the darker the better, drink slowly
    of course)
Oats
Parsley
Red Raspberry Leaf

As well, oversupply is a serious issue and can cause just as many problems. Again, please don't self-diagnose and always speak to a lactation consultant before you begin to manipulate your milk production. That said, sage is said to be excellent for slowing the flow.

A Word On Formula

There are a variety of reasons - adoption, medication, biology - that may make breastfeeding impossible. In these very rare cases (and if you are having a difficult time, please consult a lactation counselor at 1-800-LALECHE before you call it quits), it's important to honestly assess your options.

The truth is that breast is best. We all know that. So if you can access and afford human milk from a milk bank, then this should be your number one choice. Buying breast milk can be very expensive, but even using a little as a supplement to formula may go a long way in providing the plethora of benefits associated with breastfeeding. If you can't find a milk bank near you, or if banked milk is simply out of your price range, it's worth considering putting the word out. If you know somebody who's nursing it wouldn't hurt to ask, at least.

Unfortunately there's no such thing as vegan formula. Every brand available contains some sort of animal-derived ingredients, most notably vitamin D3. With that aside, you have two options: soy-based or cow's milk-based. Both of these carry their own associated benefits and risks. It's a crappy situation for a vegan to be put in, and I'm sorry.

Either way that you decide to go, you can take comfort from knowing that there are healthier choices available to you. Buying organic formula will eliminate many hormones, antibiotics, and pesticides that accumulate in conventional products. As well, check the label for unnecessary additives like high-fructose corn syrup, corn syrup solids, and cane sugar. It may be difficult to find a healthy, organic, affordable formula that fits the bill, but the search is well worth the reward.

It's frustrating that wholesome formula is so hard to find, and it's such a shame that no vegan formula exists. Still, you do the best with what you have to work with. Trust yourself to make the best choice for your child, and know that they are so lucky to have a mommy that cares so much. Babies are built out of so much more than macronutrients and minerals. It takes caring, compassion, and boundless love to put together a little person. And you, my dear, have clearly got those assets in abundance.

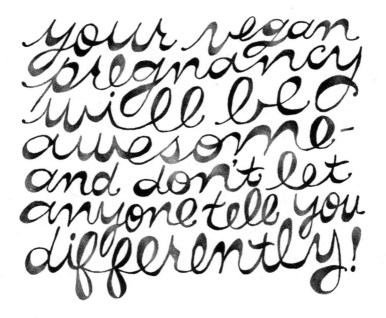

your vegan pregnancy will be awesome - and don't let anyone tell you differently!

citations

1. *Nutrition During Pregnancy.* Washington: American College of Obstetricians and Gynecologists, 2010. Print.

2. Linn, Shai, et al. "No Association between Coffee Consumption and Adverse Outcomes of Pregnancy." *The New England Journal of Medicine* 306 (1982): 141-145. Web. 29 June 2011.

3. Olshan, Andrew F., et al. "Maternal Vitamin Use and Reduced Risk of Neuroblastoma." *Epidemiology* 13.5 (2002): 575-580. Web. 29 June 2011.

4. Baily, Lynn B., and Robert J Berry. "Folic Acid Supplementation and the Occurrence of Congenital Heart Defects, Orofacial Clefts, Multiple Births, and Miscarriage." *The American Journal of Clinical Nutrition* 81.5 (2005): 12135-12175. Web. 29 June 2011.

5. Botto, Lorenzo D., et al. "Occurance of Omphalocele in Relation to Maternal Multivitamin Use: A Population-Based Study." *Pediatrics* 109 (2002): 904-908. Web. 29 June 2011.

6. "Garden of Life Vitamin D3 Derived From Lanolin." *The Vegetarian Resource Group Blog.* 29 March 2010. Web. 29 June 2011. <http://www.vrg.org/blog/2010/03/29/garden-of-life-vitamin-d3-derived-from-lanolin/>

7. "The Garden of Life Process of "Growing" Nutrients." *Garden of Life.* 2008. Web. 29 June 2011. <http://www.gardenoflife.com/vitamin-code/d3/the-garden-of-life-process-of-growing-nutrients/tabid/1901/Default.aspx>

8. American Dietetic Association. "Position Paper of the American Dietetic Association: Vegetarian Diets." *Journal of the American Dietetic Association* 109.7 (2009): 1266-1282

9. Davis, Brenda, and Vesanto Melina. *Becoming Vegan.* Summertown: Book Publishing Company. 2000. 163. Print.

10. Frasier, Abigail, et al. "Associations of Gestational Weight Gain with Maternal Body Mass Index, Waist Circumference, and Blood Pressure Measured 16 y After Pregnancy: the Avon Longitudinal Study of Parents and Children." *The American Journal of Clinical Nutrition.* 93.6 (2011): 1285-1292. Web. 29 June 2011.

11. Davis, Brenda, and Vesanto Melina. *Becoming Vegan.* Summertown: Book Publishing Company. 2000. 163. Print.

12. Davis, Brenda, and Vesanto Melina. *Becoming Vegan.* Summertown: Book Publishing Company. 2000. 162. Print.

13. Thomas, J., and F. R. Ellis. "The Health of vegans During Pregnancy." *Proceedings of the Nutrition Society.* 36.1 (1977): 46A. Web. 16 July 2011.

14. Carter, J. P., et al. "Preeclampsia and Reproductive Performance In a Community of Vegans." *Southern Medical Journal.* 80.6 (1987): 692-697. Web. 16 July 2011.

15. Fung, Teresa T. et al. "Low-Carbohydrate Diets and All-Cause and Cause-Specific Mortality." *Annals of Internal Medicine.* 153.5 (2010): 289-298. Web. 13 July 2011.

16. Davis, Brenda, and Vesanto Melina. *Becoming Vegan.* Summertown: Book Publishing Company. 2000. 164. Print.

17. Lappé, Frances Moore. *Diet for a Small Planet.* New York: Ballantine Books. 1981 (revised). 162. Print.

18. "Search the USDA National Nutrient Database for Standard Reference." *USDA Agricultural Research Service.* 2010. Web. 13 July 2011. <http://www.nal.usda.gov/fnic/foodcomp/search/>

19. Davis, Brenda, and Vesanto Melina. *Becoming Vegan.* Summertown: Book Publishing Company. 2000. 122. Print.

20. "Are Intestinal Bacteria a Reliable Source of B12?" *Vegan Outreach.* 2011. Web 13 July 2011. <http://www.veganhealth.org/b12/int>

21. Davis, Brenda, and Vesanto Melina. *Becoming Vegan.* Summertown: Book Publishing Company. 2000. 168. Print.

22. Standing Committee on the Scientific Evaluation of Dietary Reference Intakes, Food and Nutrition Board, Institute of Medicine. *Dietary Reference Intakes for Calcium, Phosphorus, Magnesium, Vitamin D and Fluoride.* Washington, DC: National Academy Press. 1997. Web. 13 July 2011.

23. Weaver, C. M., et al. "Choices for Achieving Adequate Dietary Calcium with a Vegetarian Diet." *American Journal Clinical Nutrition.* 70:3. (1999): 543S-548S. Web. 13 July 2011.

24. Massey, LK, and SJ Whiting. "Caffeine, Urinary Calcium, Calcium Metabolism, and Bone." *Journal of Nutrition.* 123:9 (1993): 1611-1614. Web. 13 July 2011.

25. Hirsch PE, and TC Peng. "Effects of Alcohol on Calcium Homeostasis and Bone." In: Anderson, John J.B. and Sanford C. Garner. *Calcium and Phosphorus in Health and Disease.* Boca Raton, FL: CRC Press. (1996): 289-300. Web. 13 July 2011.

26. Holick, Michael F, et al. "Vitamin D2 Is as Effective as Vitamin D3 In Maintaining Circulating Concentrations of 25-

Hydroxyvitamin D." *The Journal of Clinical Endocrinology & Metabolism.* 93:3 (2008): 677-681. Web. 13 July 2011.

27. Davis, Brenda, and Vesanto Melina. *Becoming Vegan.* Summertown: Book Publishing Company. 2000. 137. Print.

28. Heaney, Robert P. et al. "Human Serum 25-Hydroxycholecalciferol Response to Extended Oral Dosing with Cholecalciferol." *The American Journal of Clinical Nutrition.* 77:1 (2003): 204-210. Web. 13 July 2011.

29. Haddad, E. H., et al. "Dietary Intake and Biochemical, Hematological, and Immune Status of Vegans Compared with Nonvegetarians." *The American Journal of Clinical Nutrition.* 70:3 (1999): 586S-593S. Web. 16 July 2011.

30. Whittaker, Paul G., et al. "Iron Absorption During Normal Human Pregnancy: a Study Using Stable Isotopes." *British Journal of Nutrition.* 65 (1991): 457-463. Web. 13 July 2011.

31. Sholl, T. O., et al. "Anemia Vs. Iron Deficiency: Increased Risk Of Preterm Delivery In a Prospective Study." *The American Journal of Clinical Nutrition.* 55 (1992): 985-988. Web. 16 July 2011.

32. Cogswell, Mary E., et al. "Iron Supplementation During Pregnancy, Anemia, and Birth Weight: a Randomized Controlled Trial." *The American Journal of Clinical Nutrition.* 78.4 (2003): 773-781. Web. 16 July 2011.

33. Davis, Brenda, and Vesanto Melina. *Becoming Vegan.* Summertown: Book Publishing Company. 2000. 169. Print.

34. "Conversion Efficiency of ALA to DHA In Humans." *DHA/EPA Omega-3 Institute.* 2010. Web. 16 July 2011. <http://www.dhaomega3.org/Overview/Conversion-Efficiency-of-ALA-to-DHA-in-Humans>

35. Davis, Donald R., et al. "Changes In USDA Food Composition Data For 43 Garden Crops, 1950 to 1999." *Journal of the American College of Nutrition.* 23.6 (2004): 669-682. Web. 16 July 2011.

36. Sahakian, Vicken MD, et al. "Vitamin B6 Is Effective Therapy for Nausea and Vomiting of Pregnancy: A Randomized, Double-Blind, Placebo-Controlled Study." *Obstetrics and Gynocology.* 78.1 (1991): 33-36. Web. 17 July 2011.

37. Kristal, M. B. "Enhancement of Opioid-Mediated Analgesia: A Solution to the Enigma of Placentophagia." *Neuroscience & Biobehavioral Reviews.* 15.3 (1991): 425-435. Web. 17 July 2011.

38. Otto, S. J., et al. "Increased Risk of Postpartum Depressive Symptoms Is Associated with Slower Normalization After Pregnancy of the Functional Docosahexaenoic Acid Status." *Prostaglandins, Leukotrienes, and Essential Fatty Acids.* 69.4 (2003): 237-243. Web. 17 July 2011.

39. Hibbeln, J. R. "Seafood Consumption, the DHA Content of Mother's Milk and Prevalence Rates of Postpartum Depression: A Cross-National, Ecological Analysis." *Journal of Affective Disorders.* 69 (2002): 15-29. Web. 17 July 2011.

40. Levant, B. "N-3 (Omega-3) Fatty Acids in Postpartum Depression: Implications for Prevention and Treatment." *Depression Research and Treatment.* 2011 (2011): 16 pages. Web. 17 July 2011.

41. Jenson, Craig L. "Effects of Early Maternal Docosahexaenoic Acid Intake on Neuropsychological Status and Visual Acuity at Five Years of Age of Breast-Fed Term Infants." *The Journal of Pediatrics.* 157.6 (2010): 900-905. Web. 17 July 2011.

42. Chen, T. H., et al. "Postpartum Mood Disorders May Be Related to a Decreased Insulin Level After Delivery." *Medical Hypotheses.* 66.4 (2006): 820-823. Web. 17 July 2011.

43. Davis, Brenda, and Vesanto Melina. *Becoming Vegan.* Summertown: Book Publishing Company. 2000. 173. Print.

44. "Breastfeeding Answers from Le Leche League." *Le Leche League International.* 2011. Web. 17 July 2011. <http://www.llli.org/nb.html>

45. Davis, Brenda, and Vesanto Melina. *Becoming Vegan.* Summertown: Book Publishing Company. 2000. 172. Print.